MY MISSION TO WALK
A JOURNEY OF SIGHT, STEP, AND STRENGTH

Tonya Rabb
with Lawrence Silveira

Copyright © 2018 Tonya Rabb
All rights reserved.
ISBN: 1986709426
ISBN-13: 978-1986709422

Contents

Prologue	7
1 | Career Woman	9
2 | Georgia	29
3 | Thick White Sheet	51
4 | Back to Business School	70
5 | BLIND, Inc.	78
6 | Super Student	90
7 | Study Abroad Gone Wrong	104
8 | Paralyzed	121
9 | Norman	139
10 | Escaping Minnesota	158
11 | Professional Patient	165
12 | Getting Stronger	178
13 | Tonya's Mission to Walk	189
Epilogue	205

To my mother, for standing by my side and never letting me give up;

To Dr. Tayborn, rest in peace, for his encouragements and wisdom in teaching me how to cope with the challenges that come my way;

And finally to all of the shoulders I've stood and continue to stand upon that went the extra mile to ensure I made it through my difficult journey.

Thank you.

Prologue | Ice Cream Entrepreneur

When I was a little girl, before we moved to Chicago, my parents owned a storefront in Glen Park, Indiana called Sweet and Simple Ice Cream Parlor. Inside that ice cream joint, I inherited my business savvy: I had my first business at nine years old selling candy. It was like a little candy store inside my parents' ice cream shop and we were like the after school hangout for the children. We almost ran Dairy Queen out of business!

My dad had asked me to pick out all the candy for the kids–what the kids liked and whatnot. Reese's Pieces, Snickers, Skittles, Laffy Taffy, Nestlé Crunch, Whatchamacallits, Lemonheads, Jolly Ranchers, all of the favorites. I knew all the best ones to get. He built a little door and a little counter for me and I kinda had my own little candy shop right there inside that ice cream parlor. The whole time though, I'm not thinking he's giving me my own business, even if that was exactly what he was doing. I was just having fun helping out.

I picked out all the winning candy and he was like, "Okay now, Tonya. You collect all the money and you put it here. Here's a nickel, a dime, a penny, and a quarter rack."

And I'm thinking I'm just helping the business, right? For free. The first week, though, he came to me and he says, "Okay, this is *your* paycheck."

"Huh?"

"This is your business," he says, "and if you want to buy a thousand pieces of bubble gum, you can do it because you've earned it. But once you run out, don't ask me for anything else."

I was just like, "Independence? I can do whatever I want to with it? Oh, this rocks!"

So from that point on, since nine years old, I've always been independent–in my own strange kind of way, of course. And no matter how much has happened in my life since that little candy shop–and how much will happen in the future–I'm still just as independent as can be.

1 | Career Woman

I wanted to be a writer when I was a little girl.

My mother was an educator and, unfortunately, she was also my Kindergarten teacher. Yeah, I was like the teacher's pet and Mama's example for the rest of class, so I got teased on both sides–from the other kids *and* the teacher.

My mother would always give me extra work to do. She'd have me read, she'd have me write, she'd have me do arithmetic–I was doing flashcards since before I could hardly talk! When I was old enough to go to school, I would get the regular homework, but that wouldn't be all the work I had. I would get *extra* homework before I could go outside and play.

A lot of this extra work was reading-related. My mom would keep me busy by making me read books. She'd be like, "You don't have anything to do? Okay, go read a book." I would have to write reports on the books that I read so she knew I'd read them. She read each book before she gave them to me, too. That way, she would always know if I was joshing her or not.

 She had me typing those reports on an old-fashioned typewriter. At first, I'd feel like I was breaking my fingers on that *Murder She Wrote* kind of typewriter. I'd be like, "I can't wait until I grow up so I don't have to do this no more!" But even though I didn't like it much at first, my mom still made me write all the time. I would write letters to family members, I would write reports, and eventually, I wrote so much that I ended up liking it (but I still hated that typewriter). Because I read so much, too, I would see different patterns in how different authors wrote. All these things put together made me interested in English as a career.

 Growing up, I never stopped writing. I started writing stories. I started writing poetry. I even started helping classmates write their papers and whatnot. And so when I graduated from high school, I wanted to do something that I loved to do: write. I wanted to go to school for journalism.

 I settled on Columbia College, right there in the South Loop. When I got there, the tuition was *extremely* expensive. I think tuition was like $2,000 per quarter–I don't remember exactly–and that was over twenty years ago, so that was outrageous back then. You had students marching and everything.

 At the time I graduated from high school, my grandparents were taking care of me. Since tuition was so high, I needed financial aid, but the school said my grandfather made too much money for me to receive any support. They suggested my grandparents put their house up for a loan to send me to school. When I heard that, I said, "Oh no, you're not going to put that over my head. I'm not going to do that. I got to figure out something else to do."

I was going to get some loans myself, but I figured out I wouldn't be able to cover my student loans after I graduated with what I wanted to be. One of my professors there told me what I would probably be making for the first twenty years of my career as a journalist and I was like, "Uh, that don't add up. I ain't gonna do that."

So I dropped out of school. I wasn't going to be a writer. I had to come up with a different profession to pursue. "Well, what else do I like to do?" I asked myself.

My mom used to send me to the hairdresser every single week to get my hair done when I was younger. When I graduated from high school, though, my mom told me, "Okay, you're old enough now to pay for your own hair." She stopped sending me.

I was like, "I can't afford that." First I couldn't afford college and then I couldn't even afford doing my hair! It got me thinking though. What if I went to school to learn how to do hair professionally? Maybe I could do other people's hair and my own and I could pay my way through college without getting any loans. That's ultimately how I landed in the beauty industry. Come to find out, I loved it. It became the career for me. I wasn't gonna be a journalist. I was gonna be a cosmetologist.

So I started out doing hair. I went to school at Blue Island School of Cosmetology and I learned pretty much everything I know about doing hair there: how to do roller sets, finger waves, chemical processing, relaxers, how to use the stove, the curling irons, everything. After I graduated, I was so into all of it that my grandmother even bought me my own stove and a set of curling irons. It was a big deal. Those gifts helped me start my hair career.

    I started out working in a salon doing real soft styles like wraps and roller sets and stuff like that. Prior to me working there, though, I didn't realize you have to work with chemicals and you have to stand on your feet all day and sometimes you deal with clients who are really finicky. They can be like, "Oh, I want a flip here and this there and a cut here and a color there." Each time I had someone like that I would think, *This is just doing the most!*

    While I was doing hair in that salon, I was working for this real neat lady. Her name was Miss D. She was Italian and was always draped in gold and had her blonde hair all dolled up and drove a real nice Cadillac Allante. Oh, she was just the best. When I met her I was like, "Miss D, you really don't need this job, do you?"

    She says, "No, not really. I just love what I do."

    Everybody knew Miss D loved me to death. She called me her baby, and so then everybody would call me Miss D's Baby. She was an amazing teacher. She would always tell me, "Baby, if you ever do anything in this industry and you want to make money, specialize baby. That's where it's at. Specialize." And then every day she'd see me, she'd always say, "Specialize!" It was like she was coaxing me, giving me a mantra and cementing "Specialize!" in my head.

    But each time I heard that, I'd think, *I don't know what I want to specialize in. I just want my hair to look decent! I guess I'll see what I like.*

I decided I'd try out skincare. So one day, I went to this class out in Bensenville taught by a lady named Helma. Helma was from Germany and she had this real, real beautiful accent when she talked. When I met her, I was just sitting there in total amazement. This lady was like in her late sixties, early seventies and she was standing in front of me looking like she was only in her early forties.

"What is this? What is actually going on here?" I was completely confused! I was like, "She's lying. There's no way she can be the age she says she is."

Now here's the secret: Helma was a pioneer of the non-surgical facelift. Gold Coast Lifts and whatnot. She brought all of that to Illinois from Germany.

She told us her secret. She said, "Well, where I come from in Germany we have what are called bath houses. They're free to everyone in the community, and everyone starts getting facials there at the age of eighteen. When you start doing facials, that's when the aging stops and protects you from getting life lines."

(I call them 'life lines' because 'wrinkles' is a bad word. It's the 'W' word. We say life lines, crepey skin, W-lines, whatever, but we *don't* say 'wrinkles'. We just don't say that.)

Anyway, Helma had explained that if you get a facial every month starting at eighteen, you'll preserve your skin. You won't get life lines. But if you already have life lines, then you'll probably have to either go under the knife or do a nonsurgical face lift–that's the last attempt before you have surgery to remove them.

So I'm sitting around in the class and I'm the youngest one in the room. I was nineteen at the time. This facial stuff was real fascinating to me! There were also all these different cultures and whatnot in the class and so I started listening to other people, learning more about skin care. I was talking with everyone and I was like, "Well, how much do you charge for a facial?"

One of the ladies says, "Oh, well, I charge forty-five dollars."

I was like, "Forty five dollars and hour? Really? And you just sit down and give somebody a facial? Oh, wow, I could charge thirty-five dollars just to wash a set. And that's only an hour and a half, maybe two hours. Okay. And I'm off my feet. And I'm listening to somebody talk the whole time. I think I'd like this!"

Then it was like I heard Miss D's voice: "Specialize!"

And so I just thought this was the licks! "Specialize!" I picked skin care as what I was gonna do. I was gonna *specialize*.

I kept going back to Helma because she really knew her craft. I learned everything from nonsurgical face lifts to different facial techniques to even massage therapy. She taught a body therapy class, too, and I took it. I took all her classes. She really knew her stuff, and each time she taught me something new I was like, "Oooh!" Learning all of this about the beauty industry was addictive. So I kept coming back. I learned about body treatments, body wrapping, shea butter wraps, mud wraps, tea detoxifying wraps, you name it, I learned it. She taught me everything.

I paid for the classes out of my own pocket with money I

made doing hair, class after class after class. I took a facials class, a body treatment class, a body wrap class, nonsurgical face lift classes, aromatherapy, chemistry, European Techniques, this class, that class, all of her classes. I took every class she had and it was like so addictive.

Back then, they didn't have aesthetic licenses like they do now where you just go to school for general aesthetics. I had to take 1500 hours of different cosmetology specializations. I had like five hundred hours on the clinical floor, seven hundred and fifty hours in theory, or maybe one thousand, I can't remember. It was a lot of hours, though! And everything I was doing while in the salon counted towards my certifications. So I'm doing hair, I'm learning anatomy, I'm learning chemistry, I'm learning color theory, business, everything. It was a full program. And then if you wanted to specialize–which I did–it was even more work and even more hours. But I got the certifications. I got my cosmetology license. I learned how to do skin care, I learned how to do waxing, I learned how to do massage therapy, I learned how to do body treatments, I learned how to do it all. It was cool to me. I liked the work.

I had a hard time breaking into the spa industry after I got all this education. A lot of people just weren't educated on all the benefits and didn't want to try out what they didn't understand. And then, of course, I look a little different, my skin's a little darker, so people have a tendency to think that if you don't look like them, you don't have the skills they need. You're not on their level, even if you've got way more experience than they do. So it took a long time for me to break into that. But I did.

Eventually I rolled over to wanting to focus on massage therapy–I wanted to do so much stuff! But along the way, I'd been having problems in my marriage, and my cosmetology career kind of fell to the wayside.

But one day, my friend Lisa was hanging out with me and she says, "Tonya, it's time for you to get back into the beauty industry! You wanna do spa this and spa that. It's time!" Next thing I knew, she was driving me to a hair salon owned by a guy named Steven Deer, pushing me out of the car and yelling, "Don't come out until you get a yes!"

That wasn't the first time she'd done something crazy like that. She actually got me into the movie *Hoodlum*. One time, Lisa drove me up to a movie set and thought I should be an extra in it. She told me, "Don't come back until you get a yes from the director!"

I was just like, "Okay," totally thinking I wasn't even gonna get past security. But that was just how tenacious I was in my twenties. I got out of that car and they were shooting a scene in this building in downtown Chicago, right over by city hall. I went up to the first person I saw and asked, "Do you know where the director is?" And they pointed toward the building and so I walked that way and asked the next person I saw where the director was and then they pointed and I went and so on and so on. I just kept asking people where the director was and each person would point me a little bit closer.

Finally I got to him in this room where they're filming a dancing scene. I walked directly on up to the director, Bill Duke and I said, "Hi, how you doing?"

Now he just looked at me and everybody else was looking at me with their mouths open like in shock that I had some nerve just walking on up to the director like that, but I just kept going. "I just want to let you know I really liked your acting in *Car Wash*. I think you're a phenomenal actor. I've been in the performing arts since second grade and I know you already got this movie cast and everything, but if you have any part that's available, I would really love the opportunity to show you what I can do. If you could place me in your movie, that would be great."

Everyone's mouths just stayed dropped because I had walked right on past security to get up to him. I wasn't thinking about that at the time, I just wanted a part.

And I got one! Bill Duke looked me up and down and said, "Get costumed."

I got hired just like that! I had to wear soft finger waves, I had to get my rollers in my hair, I had to get it sprayed, all of it. I was in a nice twenties scene, swing dancing right there next to Laurence Fishburne, Vanessa Williams, Queen Latifah, all the big names in that cast. It was the scene where Vanessa Williams says, "I've heard a lot about you Bumpy Johnson." We must've heard that line a thousand times!

I guess you could say that was my acting debut, but I wanted to be behind the scenes and not really in front of the cameras, so that was the first and last time I did that.

So this time when Lisa drove me on up to Steven Deer's salon, it was like I'd been in that same position before. She told me to get out and get a job from him and the whole time I was like, "Yeah right, like he's gonna give me a chance."

His salon was in Hyde Park, Illinois right across the street from Kenwood High School—and it was one of the most popular spas at the time. It was so popular that Essence Magazine did a whole spread on it in the late nineties. The salon was this big thing, and I was worried because I didn't have much experience under my belt. It was nerve-wracking.

But I still walked in. Steven was sitting behind the counter and I said, "Are you hiring?"

He says, "What do you do?"

"I'm a skin care specialist."

"Um, yeah, come back on Tuesday. We'll get you set up."

I was so happy. He gave me that chance.

I went back out to Lisa and she says, "So…what happened?"

"He told me to come back on Tuesday," I told her.

"Yaaaaaayyyy!"

I went back Tuesday and I discovered that working there was gonna be my worst nightmare. It was gonna be that way for a good year. Reason being they already had a skin care specialist. She was seasoned and really knew her stuff, but when Steven introduced us and he said, "I want you to train Tonya," she wasn't too happy about that.

As soon as he left, the woman gave me some mean eyes. She was really mean to me, and I kinda get it now but I didn't understand it then. She told me, "I *paid* for my education and you need to pay for yours. There's no way I'm going to freely teach you what I know."

I was like, "How rude! What does she mean she doesn't want to teach me what she knows?" I thought that was very rude and mean of her, but looking back, it made sense. Why should I get the training for free when she had to go to school for it? So she forced me to go to Dermalogica, a really good skin care company, to learn about the industry. I took all their classes and learned all their different skin techniques, all their different speed waxing, all their aromatherapy, you name it, I'd done it. I got the diploma and then I finally started to train at Steven's salon.

Whenever I would work with Steven, he'd always teach me new things. Our days would start with the same back and forth. He'd call for me: "Tonya!"

Then I'd respond: "Yeah?"

"You know how to do some waxing?"

"Nope."

"Well you're gonna learn today."

I learned every day I was there, and each day it would be something different. I might come in and he'd say, "Tonya, you know how to do a body wrap?"

"Nope."

"Well you're gonna learn today."

At first I thought it was very annoying because he was harsh and really laid it on me, but he was actually mentoring me. He made sure I knew exactly what to do.

It was during his mentorship that I got my start in makeup. One day he says, "You know, Tonya. We have this big display of makeup and you come to work every day but you don't have an ounce makeup on!"

I said, "But I'm promoting beautiful skin!"

He just says, "I don't want you to come to work unless

you have on makeup."

"But it clogs my pores!"

"I will dock you every time you come into work and do not have makeup on."

So then I had to start wearing makeup. I really didn't want to at first because makeup clogs your pores. It ages you. If you don't remove the makeup properly, it can cause acne. Like, if you go to sleep with makeup on, your skin is trying to rejuvenate itself like it does every night, but the makeup clogs it up. And, just for myself, I thought I had beautiful skin without it. I've never really been hung up on my looks, but I've always thought I never really needed makeup.

What ended up changing my perspective on makeup were my clients. I didn't really like putting makeup on myself, but I loved seeing how I could transform women's faces and see the looks of pure joy when they saw how much the makeup had enhanced their looks. They would just brighten up and feel so beautiful and sexy and I really loved that part about doing makeup.

A lot of my clients who came to me for makeup ended up coming to me for skin care too because I would show them how to take care of their skin after using makeup. It helped my career quite a bit that I knew about both–I knew not only how to take care of the skin but also how to enhance their beauty with makeup.

The salon was such a beautiful place and we had some great events. Every Saturday we had trunk parties where women would walk around in really expensive lingerie. It was always very classy lingerie, like real silk robes and underwear and pajamas. The models would have their heels on, their makeup done, their hair bouncing and flowing in the wind, and the ladies who would come to the spa would watch the models and be like, "Oh, I think my husband will like this. Oh, I think he'll like that!" Sometimes we'd even have male models walking around in lingerie that the women could buy for their husbands too.

During these trunk parties, we had a receptionist who was in charge of making everything look good. Her name was Serrayah and she was *awesome*. She thought of everything. We got beautiful flowers from the florist every week that Serrayah would put around the spa. Serrayah would build out a breakfast bar every Saturday with mimosas, fruit, grapes, cherries, you name it, we had it. Little petite scones and donuts and salads–we had something for everybody. The spa would always be full and free for everyone on those Saturdays. It wasn't just a time to come in and get your hair done. It was an experience.

Steven is a very clever guy like that. Instead of people just sitting in a line and looking really mad about getting their hair done, he wanted to turn the whole spa into an experience. When you're there you have something to eat and you have nice jazz to listen to and you're getting the Steven Deer experience. People loved to come and stay all day, and that was because the salon was such a nice place.

After a while of me wearing makeup, Steven says, "Tonya!" (By now, every time I hear "Tonya" I know it's coming!) "Tonya, I've decided that every Saturday at the trunk parties, no woman leaves without makeup–and you're gonna do each and every one of their makeup *for free*."

I think, *Well what do you think this is?* But in the end, I just said, "Okay." I was still making good money.

So then I had to do makeup on other people. It wasn't just for me anymore. I wanted to learn from the makeup artist who did the spread for Essence and, of course, when I asked them I got the same spiel: "I paid for my education so you have to pay for yours. I'm not going to teach you what I know." I went to Dudley Beauty College because they had a makeup course. I learned how to blend eyeshadow really well at Dudley. I took that technique back and started doing the ladies' makeup.

I didn't really like it at first. We were an Aveda Concept Salon–meaning we sold the most popular Aveda products–so we couldn't keep the makeup on the shelves. I kept selling out, kept selling out, kept selling out. And, of course, I kept having to do more makeup.

We reached a point where I was one of Aveda's top sellers. They brought me in and were like, "What are you doing over there? All these women keep buying all this makeup and we gotta keep filling you up!" Because I was selling so much makeup, they decided to teach me more about their products, and once I started learning, I started liking doing makeup.

I guess whenever I started learning about something, I started liking it. I like learning, so when I get to learn more about hairstyling or skin care or makeup, I really start to enjoy doing those things. I learned so much about makeup in particular that I *really* liked it.

That love for makeup even took me to Hollywood. After a personal tragedy, I hopped on a plane to California and I went to Make-up Designory school (MUD) to get my journeyman's degree as a makeup artist so I could do makeup for the film industry. I got my degree to do special effects, eye fashion, stuff like that. I went from doing makeup in a salon to being a camera makeup artist for the entertainment industry. How wild is that?

I came back to Chicago right after I received my degree though. I had my daughter to think of and all her family was here. I didn't want to totally uproot her because I didn't know what my next move would be. I kinda already had a career here in Illinois within the spa industry, and then with this journeyman's degree, I was gonna come back and really be over the top. There were still lots of opportunities here in the Windy City.

I decided to open my own journeyman's studio in the West Loop where I did my makeup. Our core focus was doing makeup and skin care for the entertainment industry. It was like a whirlwind. I jumped straight into doing the makeup for calendar photo shoots–which I actually got to travel to Cancun for one of those–and I wound up doing makeup for Juan Tovar, too. He owned the "World Records" record shop in Chicago and he would put on this annual event where the store would give entertainers awards, both established artists and up-and-coming ones. And when I went, he asked me to come do makeup for the artists he managed.

That kinda put me on the map. I think that's how I ended up doing makeup for Twista and Johnny P. (More on that in a bit!) I ran into a sound engineer and he became one of my best friends because he taught me all the ropes about the entertainment industry. I'm always grateful to him for that because he was a great mentor and very instrumental to my career as a makeup artist.

But it wasn't easy breaking into the entertainment world here in Chicago, and I had some struggles before I really got going. Luckily for me, a different opportunity opened up around that time.

As I was just starting out in the entertainment industry, my old mentor Helma ("Specialize!") had decided to retire. She sold her company, HBA Aesthetics, to a guy named Robert. Robert was a very charismatic guy. He was always putting his customers first and always willing to make a deal. He had followed my career because I learned *everything* from Helma. When I got my journeyman's degree and came back to Chicago though, I was having a bit of a difficult time breaking into that makeup world. Luckily for me, Robert invited me back to HBA Aesthetics and when we met he was like, "Tonya, why don't you come teach classes for HBA Aesthetics since you know this product line better than anybody I know?"

I said, "Yeah, I could do that."

He had me teaching classes on the products, and while I'm doing all this, I'm only like twenty-five, twenty-six. The first time he put me in front of a classroom to teach, I was like, "Uh, I don't think this is gonna work." Everyone in the class was older than me. But I stepped up on the podium anyway. They all had this same blank expression on their faces, wondering what this little kid was gonna be able to teach them. I was just standing there like, "Yeah, this is going to be interesting."

So I would just jump on in, and once I really got into the

lessons, they could see that I knew my stuff. Then they were all like, "Oh, yes! You are awesome! I'm gonna come to your next class!" I would always get that initial shock factor right at first because I was so young but in the end I really did a good job.

Robert could see how well I was doing, so eventually I started setting up salons across the country, training whole staffs and doing conventions like the International Esthetics, Cosmetics, and Spa Conference (IECSC). I did a lot of travelling for HBA Aesthetics.

It was around this time when I was traveling a lot that I really began to take off as a makeup artist. My first big gig was as the key makeup artist for the video for "Pimp On" with Twista and Johnny P. It wasn't the video itself that put me on the map but who I met on set. I got on the set and I was doing the makeup for Twista and Johnny P and then all of a sudden Marshall Thompson and his wife, Tara Henderson, from the Chi-Lites were there. I don't remember why they were there. I'm not sure I even knew why back then. But it was almost like whenever there was something happening, they were there–they knew everyone! And so Tyra and Marshall were there and this was when I met them. I didn't know it then, but they would have a big influence on my makeup career. They'd give me my first big gig.

Tara and I clicked instantly. She's still one of my best friends. We would hang out a lot and she'd talk about her travels and I'd talk about my makeup and we'd just talk about all sorts of stuff. At one point, I told her, "I'm going to Vegas to do IECSC for HBA Aesthetics."

She says, "Oh, we're gonna be in L.A. around that time."

I'm like, "Really?"

Tara told me they were going on this tour for a PBS special, *70's Soul Legends*, and that Los Angeles was one of their stops. And then she asked, "You wanna come on the tour?"

I was like, "Yeah! I would love to come on the tour!"

They were supposed to appear in L.A. like two weeks before I did IECSC in Las Vegas. Tara said, "If you get to L.A., we got you."

So I flew to L.A. and joined the tour! They met me where they were filming–Universal Studios and Disneyland, of all places–and then I jumped right into doing makeup for the musicians. First I had to meet with the guy who cut all the checks for the artists and whatnot. We negotiated a bit, and then he said, "Okay, I'll give you credit as a key makeup artist."

Oh, it was awesome. That was my first big break.

So then I jumped on the rest of the tour, going with them from L.A. to San Francisco by the bay. It was absolutely beautiful there, but I was also like totally freaking out about the waterline coming right up to the Bay Bridge. When we were crossing it I was like, "Is that *water*? Like, at the same level that we're driving at? So you mean if we have an accident we're gonna drop in that?"

And they were like, "Yeah, that's water."

I said, "Oh my God."

And they were like, "Well, that's why everyone's doing eighty miles per hour across this bridge!"

I'm like, "*Oh*kay!"

We got to San Francisco safe and sound. We didn't end the tour there, though. We drove to New York, had a show there, and then we went to Philly. When we got to Philly all the artists who were a part of that PBS special were there, and it was really exciting for me because I got to do all of the makeup on the set, all the makeup for all the major R&B groups from the '70s. The Stylistics to the Chi-Lites to Harold Melvin's Blue Notes to Cuba Gooding Sr. and even the host, JJ from *Good Times*–I did all of their makeup. I'm so thankful for that tour because they were major instruments in my career, and they were great people too! They'd always call me "Baby Girl" because I looked so young. I was Baby Girl to all the crew.

And then just like that, when I was done doing makeup for them in Philly, they paid for my ticket and flew me back to Vegas for the convention. I don't think I'll ever forget that tour. They had opened the door for me. After that, my career took off. I was in demand everywhere I went.

I did calendars, worked with master cosmetologists, traveled all over the place, I did makeup for a student film called *Isolation*, and I also did music videos, like the one did with Twista and Johnny P. The last video I did was a music video with Gucci Mane. The song's called "Icy". I did all the makeup for the women in the video. I had an infatuation with Aaliyah's makeup artist at the time because he had such creative work with the shimmer, the pop, the iridescence, all of it. I took on that same bubblegum look and whatnot for the "Icy" video.

My mom fussed at me when she saw it. You know how moms do with all that hip-hop, that rap. "Tonya," she said, "you need to do something of higher caliber. It is nice, though, your makeup." I thought I did a good job. She just didn't like the song's message I guess.

Once my career took off, it was like everybody wanted me to work for them. Makeup, cosmetology, massage therapy, everything I did, people wanted me to do. And so as my career continued to grow, I moved to Atlanta, Georgia. Why? Because I worked for all the top spas in Chicago and I felt like I had reached my pinnacle. It's really hard to make it in Chicago as a professional and so if you can make it in the Windy City, you can make it anywhere. I wanted a change. I grew up here, my husband grew up here, and everywhere I went I had memories. I just wanted to do something different, something fresh. And I would've gone back to L.A., but I thought if I went there it would've been too fast-paced to raise a child. So I moved to Atlanta, the Hollywood of the South.

Looking back, California might've been better than Atlanta. Who would've thunk?

2 | Georgia

I got married at eighteen, had a beautiful daughter at nineteen, and became a widow at twenty-four.

We were high school sweethearts, Robert and I. I practically grew up with him. We were like brother and sister almost, always getting into mischievous things. One time we stole his mom's car together! He was like, "You steer it and I'll push!" We pushed it out of the driveway and then we started the engine up and went. We were always doing crazy things like that. He was my best friend. We could complete each other's sentences, and at eighteen, we were married.

One year later and I had my daughter, Mona Sha'e. She was beautiful–a bundle of joy. But it was a little scary, too, because she looked exactly like me. You know how babies don't look like anybody when they're first born? Well, Sha'e wasn't like that. She looked exactly like me.

We used to talk to her when she was still inside me and so she recognized our voices right after being born. When they put her on my chest, she opened those little eyes and looked up at me. Her dad was like, "Hey!" and she looked over at him like, "I know that voice!"

She was a definitely a bundle of joy. Very alert, very smart, very bright. She still looks like me.

We were a happy little family, but then right before my twenty-fifth birthday, Robert died abruptly in a car accident. It was heartbreaking for me. I remember he would always tell me, "Ooh, I can't wait until you turn twenty-five. You gonna be a heartbreaker!" But he never got to be there for my twenty-fifth.

His car had flipped over. The paramedics tried to save him, but he was on life support and it wasn't looking good. He was still fighting for his life, but I think deep down I knew this would be the last time I saw him. When he was on some of his last breaths, I made a promise to him. "Don't worry about Shay," I told him. "I'm gonna take care of her for you and me both."

It was a lot to process. I could see tears running down his eyes like he could hear me, but he had a tube running down his throat. The doctor said that if he lost his coughing response, that would be it.

I had to go lie down. I stayed there in the hospital and lay down in the waiting area for intensive care. I used to always have this thing where I would sleep with the cover over my face, so I put the coat I was wearing over my head just like a sheet and I slept.

When we were married, Robert would always have this habit of standing over me and watching me sleep. I could always feel his presence whenever he did that. This particular time while I had the coat over my head, I was laying down and I felt this real cold presence come into the room. Now, hospitals are always cold, but this was different. It felt like Robert was standing there.

I heard his voice. "Tonya," he said. "Don't be afraid to let me go."

I couldn't believe it. I was like, "What? No no no no no, I don't believe that. Robert's a fighter!"

I threw the coat off my face and I ran toward his room and when I got there, the nurse was standing right outside the door. He was on the phone with the doctor. His back was turned–he didn't see me come up–and then I heard him say, "He just lost his coughing response."

I started freaking out and crying. I was there all by myself. The nurse heard me and turned around. He was like, "Oh no no no, Miss Rabb, no please. I'm so sorry. You didn't hear that from me, Miss Rabb."

Nurses are not supposed to deliver the news. The doctors are the ones who do that. But for some reason, Robert's spirit had told me he was making the transition and I had to go see for myself. I'd walked up on the nurse while he was telling the doctor. He just kept trying to calm me down. "No no no no, please calm down, Miss Rabb. Do you want us to call you a chaplain?"

I really started freaking out then. I didn't want to say goodbye.

I forced myself back to the waiting room and called Robert's family and told them to get there right away. They weren't there already because of all the days it could've been, it was Memorial Day. They rushed to the hospital, and when Robert's father came, I said, "I don't know what I'm gonna tell Mona Sha'e. This is gonna break her heart and I don't know how to deliver this to her."

She was a real daddy's girl. I didn't have the strength to figure out how to tell her. I was just freaking out and crying and Robert's dad really comforted me. He told me, "Don't worry. I'll take care of it for you."

He went home that day and everyone was crying and he went upstairs to my daughter. She hadn't seen her father in a few days since he'd been admitted to the hospital and she was like, "Where's my daddy?" He put her on his lap and told her that her dad wasn't coming home anymore. I will always be appreciative of him for that because I was too weak to do it myself.

Robert had told me a few days before the accident, "Oh Tonya, I've decided to be an organ donor!"

I was like, "Oh no no no, don't do that."

I had spent a bit of time in a nursing program before settling on my cosmetology career. In that program my teacher told us to never sign up to be a donor because if you do, doctors won't always try everything to save your life since your organs are important and there are people in line who need them. While you're still alive and fresh, they can take your organs and give them to the next person in line. That sounded kinda jaded but it was just the brutally honest truth. And so when he told me that he'd decided to be an organ donor, I was like, "Oh no, you should take that off your drivers license."

He told me, "Well, I don't want to be a vegetable if anything were to happen to me. I'd rather my organs go to a good use."

I get it. I really get it *now*! But because he was an organ donor, I don't think they did everything they could to try to save him. They were like, "Well, we're gonna go ahead and take his organs."

I was like, "No no no no, do everything you can to save him first." They decided to take the tube out of his mouth and see if he woke up on his own. If he didn't, then they were just gonna take his organs. And he didn't wake up on his own.

To this day I think I should have been in there with him. They wouldn't allow me in there to see if he woke up and could speak on his own. To see if he might've had a chance. That's always a question that's been at the back of my mind. I don't think I'll ever get rid of it.

It was all very traumatizing. I realized I had to kick it up a notch because I was the sole breadwinner for my daughter, and I had to be both mother *and* father. I had to focus on my daughter, and so I didn't really get a chance to mourn properly. My remedy to my mourning was to work until I dropped. Work work work work work. Always working. Try to do something constructive with it. I ended up mourning him for a good ten years that way, never fully able to let that grief go.

At one point while I was pursuing my makeup career, I decided I needed some guidance. There was a lot going on emotionally and I ended up landing at this church called Word of Faith. It wasn't the church I usually went to.

I was working at the time and I always worked weekends

so I couldn't make it to my usual church on Sundays. That was fine by me because I'd been listening to the words since I was born! I'm from a family of pastors, of course I knew it all! But I think everybody still needs some kind of spiritual guidance to keep them balanced in life, and so I made sure to go after work each day and pay my tithes, even though I couldn't make it to the services. The pastor there, Pastor Hinkel, kept noticing that I would come straight after work just to pay my tithes, and so one Sunday I'm paying my tithes and he says, "I know you can't make the service here on Sundays, so this is what I want you to do. I want you to go to this other church in the evenings and I think you'll get the words you need."

So I went to this other church's evening service, and I found out my friend Lisa went there too, so I started going with her. Now, Dr. Singleton, the pastor at Word of Faith, had a different way of giving the words. He would teach directly out of the bible but he would also put a story to it. He would relate the messages to everyday life, and he always had the greatest sense of humor to go with his sermons. Some of the things he'd say would just make me so tickled and I would laugh and laugh! I'd never done that before at church. I could actually relate to this pastor.

He always taught prosperity, too. He and his sermons were a big influence in my life. He had this sermon where he kept preaching this series, "What Do You Have In Your Hand." He'd be like, "Well, God wants us to be entrepreneurs. What do you already have in your hand? Every job you work, you should take its experience and use those skills to the fullest. Apply them to whatever business you want to open one day because God wants you to be prosperous so you can help other people and be a good steward. You shouldn't just be wealthy so you can be totally selfish and see how many cars or how many rooms in a house you can get. God wants us to be entrepreneurs."

There were a lot of people who were go-getters at Word of Faith, so I not only connected with the message but I connected with the people. I really enjoyed going to this church and I really enjoyed listening to the lessons. I really took to his lessons, especially the one about how God wants us to be entrepreneurs, probably because I'd been entrepreneurial for as long as I can remember.

Now, throughout my whole life, I kept trying to start businesses. And I kept failing! I think my only successful business venture was my candy store, and that was only because my parents made sure I was successful at that one! I'd want to open spas and beauty studios and other businesses in the beauty industry, but where I had talent when it came to facials and makeup and massage, I just didn't have that same talent on the administrative side. I kept failing at the business part of business. So I when I came to Word of Faith, I said, "You know what, I'm not going to try one more ounce of what I've always done." I didn't just want to jump into another business with no knowledge on it. I wanted to learn! So I'd go to people and I'd ask, "Can you mentor me? Can you show me how to do this?" And then I'd get the same spiel I always got: "Well, I'm not going to give you everything I know when I paid for my education. You've gotta go get yours too." So practically everything I've done for my career, I had to pay my way. I had to go to school. And it was the same when I got to Atlanta.

I didn't jump right into business school, though. This is what happened. I was working at Elizabeth Arden in Chicago and I went to a family reunion in Atlanta, Georgia. I was already thinking about moving at this time. I wanted to get away from all the memories I had with my husband in Chicago. And so while I was in Atlanta, I fell in love with the green grass and the blue sky and just how beautiful everything was. I decided that I was gonna move there.

"I'm gonna find me a job working down here," I said. "I ain't never had problems finding jobs and so let me find a job while I'm down here."

I went to this salon spa where Whitney Houston and her daughter Bobbi were featured going to in Alpharetta, a suburb just north of Atlanta. I forget what the name was, but I went in and I talked to the owner of the spa and he just totally fell in love with my career and everything. He said, "Oh, we can use you. We can bring you in as our Head Aesthetician."

Now, Elizabeth Arden wasn't giving me a Head Aesthetician position. They wanted me to just be a manager over the massage therapy and whatnot because I had a high number of returning clients, but I didn't want that position. So I told the owner, "Well, uh, I could do that. I could totally do that."

And so I moved. I didn't have them sign a contract about them paying for my moving expenses or anything like that, even though I probably should have. I moved with no problem–I wanted to move anyway–but I had never met the owner's wife. She was pregnant (and so also probably a little hormonal). When I finally met her, she was like, "Who are you? And what are you doing? Oh, you think you're going to be our Head Aesthetician?"

I said, "Well, I'm here. I've been in the industry for like fifteen years and I can build out your aesthetic department and this that and the other." She still wasn't having it, though. "You might want to discuss this with your husband."

Turns out, they already had a Head Aesthetician and she wasn't going for me being there. The wife and the Head Aesthetician were in cahoots together. We just didn't get along. I thought I could make good sales, but the husband told me, "Well, Tonya, you know I really like you, but I love my wife and I gotta go with what my wife says. She's pregnant, you know, and so we have to let you go."

I was like, "Let me go! After fifteen hundred dollars of my own money! Are you serious!?" So I was out of a job.

It really started to hit me. I just up and moved everything. Uprooted my whole life. I was like, "Oh my God, what am I gonna do?"

I had to hustle. I did some bartending (I'd done bartending before in Chicago), I was working part time at a spa called Juve The Spa, I was working at a salon just for men called Executive Barber Salon, I was doing wraps and facials and massage therapy and I was just always working. Working working working. And because of it, I couldn't spend as much time with my daughter as I wanted to. She was becoming a latchkey kid and I didn't like that. It really broke my heart.

So I made a plan. I was like, "Okay, Sha'e, this is what

we're gonna do. I'm gonna send you home to Chicago with Grammy for the summer, Mommy's gonna re-up on money, and then I'm gonna bring you back in the fall for school."

But she didn't come back that fall. Sha'e was at school in a nice area with a lot of wealthy kids and whatnot, but when she went to see Grandma for the summer, Grandma convinced Sha'e to stay in Chicago and go to school there for the year.

Of course I wasn't happy about that. I just started moping around because I was used to dragging my daughter around with me everywhere I went. I got so mopey that at one point one of my friends called me to talk some sense into me. She said, "Tonya! Listen to me. Now you stop that moping."

"But what am I gonna do? My daughter's not here, I'm here all by myself, and blah blah blah, woe is me."

She was not gonna let me keep this sadness up. "This is exactly what you're gonna do," she said. "You're gonna quit moping and crying and doing all this sad stuff and you're gonna get your butt up and you're gonna go sign yourself up for college and you're gonna get yourself a degree! Do you hear me? Some people don't even have anyone to take care of their kids and you're sitting up here fussing about what you're gonna do. Quit moping and go to school and get around some good people."

That was the push I needed. "Yeah, I guess that's what I'll do," I said. "You know what, I think I wanna own a resort one day, and it's gonna cost millions of dollars to do this. I'm gonna have to know how to pay back the people who give me this money and know how to manage the business, so I might as well go to school for business and accounting!"

I was finally gonna do the business thing. I was gonna follow Dr. Singleton's sermon and learn how to be an entrepreneur.

I started going to Herzing University, right across the street from Lennox Mall (at the time). When I got there, I wasn't really sure if I wanted to do it or not. It was a little scary.

But then I heard this teacher speak and he was so inspiring. The odds were against me going to this school: I had no experience in business, I was older than most of the students, and I was still scared I might fail. But the professor kept speaking and kept speaking and kept speaking and he was really inspiring. His name was Mr. Breelin. He talked about how you've got to follow your life's destiny and how you're here for a purpose and a reason and how you've got to follow your dreams and get a good education so you can make a difference in other people's lives. It was a bunch of stuff like that.

After hearing him speak, I was like, "Okay, that's it, I'll sign up for school." It wasn't the school, it was *him*.

The technique that Herzing used wasn't like the average college technique. It was more of a guerrilla style, really hands-on. Oh, it was phenomenal. You could go take a class and instantly apply what you learned to your business.

I loved Herzing because I could take a course in Excel and immediately apply what I learned to my business and do my spreadsheets. I could take a class in marketing and I could learn about how businesses were structured through that. I could take the knowledge I gained and I could apply it to pretty much anything I wanted to do with business and marketing. I was able to apply everything I learned. It was all real-time, too. It wasn't like I had to wait until I graduated. You take a class and you apply it to your business the very next day.

I took accounting, I took business management, I took speech, I took writing, I took Excel, Word, PowerPoint, I took computers, I took all of them. One of the first classes I took that really got me excited for school was Critical Thinking. Mr. Breelin actually taught that class. That was pretty cool. I took psychology, too. That was one of my hardest courses. I took business law–learned how to write contracts and whatnot. I would also take extra classes that weren't necessarily in my major like Time Management because I thought they could help enhance me as an overall student. You name it, I took it.

That's how I got into the Atlanta Black Chamber of Commerce. They had lots of organizations there–Toastmasters, too! They would teach you how to speak and change your voice to match what you were saying and how to get the arms out and moving so you're not so rigid, you know? And in all these organizations, you were dealing with people. They taught you how to interact with people, how to market yourself.

I loved how real-time Herzing was because I was working for myself as well. I managed to pick up a part time job at Spa on Paces where all my appointments would be after school from five to eight. On Saturdays, I'd work in the spa all day.

Spa on Paces was a unique place because a lot of celebrities came there. It was a very private boutique spa in the heart of Buckhead. That's where a lot of celebrities live in

Georgia. The spa was hidden away in its own little cul-de-sac so high-profile people didn't have to worry about fans rushing in on them and being like, "Oh my God! Can I get an autograph?" They could all just come on in, get their service, and then go quietly.

I met a lot of people at that spa–Demi Moore, Jill Scott, to name a few–and everyone was extremely nice. I'm gonna go off topic for a second, but one of my favorite stories from there was when I met Ellen DeGeneres. She came in with her girlfriend and she was so bubbly. I looked at her because I couldn't quite tell if it was really her, and she knew that I knew she looked familiar but couldn't quite register. Eventually I said, "Man, you look familiar!"

She just says, "Oh girl, yeah, I hear that all the time. People say I look like Ellen DeGeneres."

"Oh, oh okay." I thought she was serious! I thought she was just saying that she looked like Ellen DeGeneres! Come to find out, it really *was* her. We were doing a couple's massage and she was cracking jokes the whole time–that's when I realized it was her. I was just thinking, *Can you believe this woman, telling jokes this whole time? She is hilarious!* She was just as bubbly, just as personable as she is on TV.

And when she left, she left a real handsome tip, too. Meeting Ellen was definitely one of the highlights from my time at Spa on Paces.

So anyway, I'm going to school and I'm doing really well. I kept a routine because I never ever wanted to fall behind in my work. I wanted to keep my GPA up. I'm passing my classes, earning money at the spa, and I'm making friends. I'm always positive with my classmates, too. I'd be like, "How's it going?" If they would have an attitude like, "Girl, look–" I wouldn't let them go no further. I'd be like, "Okay, you gotta pay that back with interest."

They'd say, "Okay, Tonya. Yeah, I gotta get off my game. You right." Encouragement is important. I would always try to encourage my peers.

One of my professors took note of how friendly I was with all the other students. Dr. Kevin Laurent was my tutor for accounting and he would watch how I interacted with my peers, encouraging everyone and whatnot. He came to me one day and said, "Hey, Tonya! I think you would do good in politics."

"Nah, I ain't no politician."

And then I walked off. I didn't want nothing to do with politics.

But he came back, and he kept coming back. He just kept coaxing me every time he saw me. "Okay," he'd say. "Well, maybe I was wrong about politics, but don't you care about your student body and your friends?"

"Yeah, I do, but I don't know nothing about politics." And I would just keep walking.

Finally one day he trapped me. I was supposed to go to China for a study abroad trip, but had I gone on the trip, I would've missed my daughter's eighth grade graduation. I turned down China to go see my daughter graduate in Chicago. And so because I didn't go, the president of the Future Business Leaders of America went to China instead, and that left her spot in the organization open.

Well, it turned out that Dr. Laurent was the professor who was in charge of the Future Business Leaders of America. When the president took my spot on the study abroad trip, Dr. Laurent was like, "Tonya, you know the president is gone."

I was real suspicious, because I don't want to be a part of the FBLA. I said, "Yeah, I know she's gone."

He asked, "Well, can you stand in her place?"

"I don't know the first thing about being a president!"

"Tonya, I'll walk you through it."

And so after a little more coaxing, I accepted the position, not knowing he was actually setting me up to replace her permanently. I thought it was just gonna be a temporary thing.

When I became president of FBLA, Dr. Laurent helped guide me a little bit, but I still didn't know the first thing about being in charge. I was like, "Okay, so what am I supposed to do? Hmm. Well, I'm gonna go get an expert!"

Around that time I had just finished reading *The Covenant with Black America* by Tavis Smiley. It was a pretty good book. It was all about economics and how to build the economy and be entrepreneurs and it was just really uplifting to me. So one day I saw an advertisement for a panel in connection with the book. I was like, "Okay, I think I'll go."

When I got there and saw all the people involved, I realized I could connect these people to FBLA. There was a bunch being said about economics and that was right up my alley, being a business administration and accounting student.

One of the people there was Michael Hill, the president of the Atlanta Black Chamber of Commerce (AMBCC) and he was on the panel. I sat there in the audience listening to him talk about how we should put our monies together and reestablish our communities and like business this and entrepreneurship that and I was just like, "Yeah, he's the one! I need him to come in and speak to Herzing's FBLA." I got his information and left the event.

The next day, I called him. He kinda blew me off, like, "Yeah yeah yeah, okay, no thanks."

So I called him again. No response. I left a message.

I called him again and again and again. Never any answer. Finally, I was just like, "Look, Mr. Hill. This is Tonya Rabb. I've left several messages and I'm really interested in having you come speak at my school because I'm president of Herzing's Future Business Leaders of America branch and I think your influence could help our student body transfer over to a successful career and become successful entrepreneurs. I need someone to mentor and help groom this organization because I don't have the experience, but I know you do."

I finally got a call back.

"How old are you?" he asked. I told him how old I was and he said, "I like your tenacity. I'll come meet with you."

So he came and met with me at the school and in order for him to speak with the other students and whatnot, I had to get permission from the president of the school. But when he and I asked, the school was like, "Wait a minute. Why don't you partner with us?"

He said, "Well, the only way I'll do a partnership with your school is if you let Tonya be the liaison."

So not only did I get the AMBCC President to come speak to the FBLA, but he also gave me a liaison role with his organization! It was awesome!

When the partnership first began Michael asked me, "Tonya, what do you want out of this?"

I was still green behind the ears and said, "I just want everyone to graduate and have a successful career and that they're able to move upward and make a difference. I just want to make a difference!"

He was like, "Yeah, but what's in it for *you*?"

"That's what's in it for me," I said. "I just want to make a difference."

So I became Herzing's liaison for the Atlanta Black Chamber of Commerce. I would go to Herzing every Saturday and open up one of the classrooms for classes that professionals from the AMBCC would teach each weekend. We would teach people how to manage their money, how to get a checking account, how to make a budget, how to market yourself, how to network, how to plan for conventions and campaigns, how to do pretty much anything someone in business would need to know. AMBCC was a resource for people who were in the business world: small business owners, new entrepreneurs, people who just wanted to start a business. Anyone and everyone was welcome.

AMBCC really helped the Herzing students. They'd have projects where they would connect people with different projects and different businesses and sometimes they would take people and give them internship opportunities in major corporations. They'd link small businesses with bigger businesses and they would have events with like NASCAR and McDonalds and St. Jude's Children Hospital just to really get people out there and learning. It was a really awesome experience. It was wild.

To this day, the Atlanta Black Chamber of Commerce is still partnering with Herzing. The partnership worked so well that the student body really started to like me. In fact, they liked me so much they elected me president of Student Government Association as well.

I was only president for two or three weeks though. Everyone wants to be president. Everyone's fighting for that position. They were all complaining about me being president for two organizations, both FBLA and SGA, so I had to step down from one of them. I chose SGA. They hurried up and got me out of that position.

Even though I was only in the position for a short time, I did have one accomplishment. I brought the students in for a panel and asked them what we could do to improve Herzing. I really genuinely cared for the students and the student body, and I wanted to know what we could do to make them more successful. We talked about credit hours, we talked about funding, we talked about all the issues. Herzing didn't really like that, though. They thought I should have been framing it differently. They were like, "You're here for us, not for them."

I was livid. So that kinda hastened my leaving that president position. They told me, "Tonya, we know you're very popular and you keep your GPA up and everything, but we think you should step down from one of your positions, either Student Government Association or the Future Business Leaders of America. You can still be a *part* of SGA, we just prefer you not hold two positions as president. It's a conflict of interest." So I left SGA as president and stayed on as like Vice President or something. I don't remember. I was still a part of the organization though.

My daughter came back home during my second year at Herzing once I'd finally gotten settled there. When she would go to school, I'd be at school, too, so it wasn't too difficult to be there for her, but it was still another responsibility to add to my plate. I was starting to get busy!

Herzing had all these great workshops, and one of them was on time management. I would follow everything I learned to a T and it really helped me in school.

I had great time management. I had everything down to a routine. I would go to school from nine to eleven, and then I stayed on campus to get my homework done. I told Spa on Paces that I didn't get out of school until five o'clock so I could get all my homework done the same day I was issued it. The spa wasn't going to call me and disrespect my time for school. So that's how I kept my GPA up. And then at Spa of Paces, I would go in from six to eight, Monday through Friday, and then all day Saturday, the owner and I would hold it down together. We'd do appointments back to back all the way to close on Saturday. I made good money, but I had to see a lot of people for that to happen.

Sundays were my favorite day. Sunday was Mommy & Daughter Day. Sha'e and I would go do whatever we wanted to do on those days. And we *always* had Mommy & Daughter Day on Sundays no matter what—even when she was a little girl and we lived in Chicago. I would take her to parks or we would go out for breakfast and get these big huge pancakes and omelets that I would spend so much time cutting up for her first, and by the time I'd get to my food it'd be cold. I would take her to plays, or we would play dress up to look like each other, or we'd go to the movies and see something fun. I was always teaching her about facials and waxing and stuff, too, because that's what I did. She was a real prima donna!

When I had everything balanced out and my time all managed nicely, I would take on projects like video shoots and whatnot because I had earned my stripes as a makeup artist and I wanted to keep that going too. I could call my shots on what I wanted to do and when I wanted to do it. That was like a little side gig, though.

As I did all the above, I told myself I had to get A's in my classes. So I would push myself. If I wasn't getting an A, I wasn't going to treat myself. But when I would get my A's, then I had some fun. I would go to my favorite place called Churchill Grounds, which was right next door to Fox Theatre on Peachtree Street. It breaks my heart that it's no longer there. But Churchill Grounds was my escape because you would go in and it'd just look like a little café. You'd have desserts and sweets in this little bakery over to the side and if you wanted to get something to eat you could. Then you have a guy standing at a curtained door. You'd pay your admission to get in and you'd go through that curtain and see the stage sitting right there in front of you. You have little round cocktail tables to sit at, almost like in *Casablanca*, and if you were VIP there was a section with couches all around and a curtain around it. There was a bar where you could order drinks and if you wanted more than just what you got from the bakery, you could order dinner too. And then finally you'd sit down with your dessert and your drink and get ready for the performance.

They had *jazz*. Every night of the week. They had acid jazz, women's jazz, classical jazz, all sorts of jazz. It was a different theme every night, each of the seven days of the week, and so I would always go there to treat myself. I'd get my favorite Port wine, my favorite dessert, every once in a while some dinner, too, and I'd sit there and just listen. That was my escape. I would have a good time.

I loved that place because it was a cool setting, but also because I really love jazz—the acoustic sound, the creativity, the instruments. Oh, the instruments! You've got the flute, you've got the piano, you've got the base, you've got the violin, you've got the drums, you've got all this live music going on at one time just going off the feel of each other. I started playing by reading sheet music, but with jazz it's different because they're not looking at a playbook. They're just playing. Someone starts off and someone else jumps in and they're all ad-libbing but it all sounds good. It just all comes together and sounds so beautiful. When you listen to music nowadays, a lot of it is electronic, computerized. It's nothing like hearing live music. To hear the natural sound coming from live music—it's magic.

I had a *lot* going on, with school, with FBLA and SGA, with working in the spa, with spending time with my daughter, with everything. I never really had time for me, other than the few times I treated myself to a night of jazz. I would just work until I drop. Work work work work. I would work so much so I wouldn't have to think about my husband. So I wouldn't have to mourn. I don't think that was healthy. I did this for ten years straight.

When I woke up the morning after my 35th birthday, I guess my body was ready to tell me that it had had enough of that always-working lifestyle. It was ready to tell me that I needed to slow down.

3 | Thick White Sheet

During my time in Atlanta, I went to this place called Sapelo Island. I'd been really stressed out and really overwhelmed and so Mr. Breelin came to me and said, "You should come onto this couple's retreat with me and my fiancé."

I thought that was a little weird. "But I'm not in a couple," I told him.

"It'll be a healing experience for you. Come on."

He told me about Sapelo Island and it sounded like a relaxing, refreshing place. I decided to go. I was the only one on this couple's retreat by myself; Mr. Breelin and his fiancé were there along with two other couples. I was like a seventh wheel I guess you could say, but in a sense, I was comfortable. I know that sounds crazy, but I was really comfortable by myself. It was like a healing experience for me because I was able to collect seashells on the beach, write poetry, walk around in all the nature, and just be so, so peaceful.

We took a ferry over to the island because that was the

only way to get there. Doves flew along the boat, welcoming us to the island. Oh, it was so beautiful, right from the start. And it just kept getting better.

Everything was just totally peaceful. The seafood is straight from the ocean, there are live chickens walking around, there are all kinds of different birds chirping in the trees, wild boars just walking along the side of the roads, alligators in the ponds with no fences around them or nothing. It was just beautiful, peaceful, quiet.

Mr. Breelin had a direct connection to Lula and George, two of the people who lived on the island. Lula and George gave tours of the island because they were direct descendants of who had lived there in the past. They were like a team. George would lead the tours where we'd hop in the back of this pick-up truck and ride around the island. He'd stop for gas at the island's only gas pump and take us to the trailers we stayed in, he'd take us to the Reynolds Mansion–this real beautiful mansion built in the early 1800's from cowrie shells, lime, and sand–he'd take us around the ponds and the landscaping and the gardens over by all the living quarters, he'd take us by the barn where slaves were sold way back when, he'd take us over to the forest preserve with all of its nature and flowers and all the green, and then he'd take us to the beachfront. We actually got to go out to the beachfront at night! Oh my God, it was so beautiful. You'd see the sky and all the stars and that's when I would collect my cowrie shells. When the couples were relaxing, I'd stay out of their way and collect the shells to bring home with me.

And when it was time to eat, we went to Lula's Kitchen.

All of the presidents up to that point—and I'm talking about the presidents of the *United States*—would visit the island and eat at Lula's Kitchen. That's how good Lula's food was. And oh boy was it good! George has this shack outside of the house where he cooks his seafood and throws it all in one big stock pot and stirs it up real good. It's almost like a smokehouse, like it's so small that only two people can fit inside. The last night we ate, they had everything—shrimp, chicken, fish, steak, biscuits, greens, desserts, the whole nine, all freshly made, too. It was just so good that I wanted to stay forever. I even told them that too! I was like, "Lula, I promise you, I'll work for free if you could just let me live here with you and feed me all of your delicious food. I *love* this place."

She was so sweet, she was like, "Well sweetie, you just come on back anytime. You have an open invitation."

We were there for a whole week, and when we left, I watched the doves say goodbye to us the same way they had welcomed us. I was so inspired by the trip, I wrote a poem called "My Special Place" while I was on the island.

<u>MY SPECIAL PLACE</u>

Let me tell you about a place I know

Once I am finished painting this picture of my special place
In your mind you would actually want to go

To escape into Peace, Calmness and Serenity
Seems to be where I am

To leave the hustle and bustle behind
To continue the never ending journey
For me in which I want to find

The welcoming of the sea gulls gliding and soaring through in a gentle way
with so much freedom and peace
As if they were ancestors from before
Granting me with mental telepathy
To have a beautiful journey

You might be thinking of a destination with five star accommodations
Instead, I am talking of a place and time so profound

I am grateful at this point and time
This is where I am supposed to be

Not a five star hotel
But instead something a whole lot better

I found Serenity and Peace,
Which will help me to continue the journey
Of knowing and becoming a leader myself
In turn help others to lead nations

The air of this place is so crisp and clean
The breeze of the trees are so soft and welcoming
The sound of the music of the birds is so loving and inviting

Knowing the fact that I have to leave and return
Is something in my mind and soul I am fighting

The world here is much like it should be
Away from the cares of the materialistic,
Dominant, cold and self-preserving society
Instead it's filled with Love, Peace and Serenity
Now that's an excellent variety

It's much like the beautiful seashells along its beautiful shore with different characters, shades of colors

The feel of the smooth or roughness and
The shapes and character

Being different in their own way
Without worrying about the rest of
The world's existence

Instead, each shell has a different story to tell
In how they came to be
Molded into the shell they are
This is my most spiritual place by far

Even in the calmness of the night
The horizon is so amazingly round,
As a sphere filled with nothing but
Beautiful stars

To the point it actually proves the theory
The earth is round
When I think of this place
I marvel at the peace I have found

At My Special Place
You have the comfort of home
With the best cooked meals
That you can tell were slowly prepared
With care and lots of love
Ruth's Chris,
No not even they can top these meals
There is nothing above
Go back to the real world
Why should I want to go there?
Where there is not enough love and peace everywhere

Seeing nature for its beautiful, peaceful state in which it really exists

Makes me fall in love with this atmosphere
And to think of parting from this place makes me not want to leave and let go
Instead, I really want to resist

In this place,
Where I lay my head down to sleep
It is so warm, comfortable, and secure
I feel like a little girl once again
Without a care in the world

Although, waiting on the other side of my special place
Is the COLD, HARSH, CONFUSED, DEFIANT WORLD
Filled with so much HATE, UNCONCERN, GREED, AND
SURVIVAL BY ANY MEANS NECESSARY

I have grown up to experience and SEE
In that world I am like Tupac said,
As an adult, I AM
That Rose that Grew out of Concrete
Not easily too and won't except defeat

Once again, I LOVE MY SPECIAL PLACE
Away from the minute things like, WORRY, CONFUSION,
POLITICS and CARES OF MATERIALISTIC THINGS
That are so trivial

I thank the universe and ancestors for allowing me the rite to write this verse
All that should exist is Love
And unbalance the scale without hate
I know this realm would be a better place

I think we could all relate
All I know is Love is My Special Place

Where it conquers over hate
When it's standing face to face

Because I know this is something and somewhere

I would not want to leave or let go

Such a place I describe
Does it really exist for real or
Is it all in my mind?

If it's possible, I bet you would really want to know
And if it is, I am sure you would want to go.

The retreat was like totally amazing–the most peaceful thing I've ever experienced in my life. If I could have just stayed on that island, stayed in all that serenity for the rest of time, I would have. It was perfect.

Because two weeks later, I lost my eyesight, and it felt like I had left my spirit on Sapelo Island.

+

It was my 35th birthday. I woke up in the morning and everything was just ghostly white. I was like, "Hm. Okay. Um, maybe I just need to lie down and go back to sleep. Maybe I just partied a little too hard." I usually have a limit of two drinks when I go out but I think I had three for my birthday. I thought that was why I couldn't see. I just figured I needed to lie back down and go to sleep and it would be okay. It would just go away.

I woke up again and everything was still ghostly white. I couldn't understand it. I was definitely in denial. I said, "Wow. Well, um, okay. Maybe I'm just having a bad day and I need to take it easy." It just didn't seem like it was possible. I couldn't see anything. This wasn't happening. I was just like, "Okay, this is only temporary. I'll be better by tomorrow. I just need to rest through the day and take it one day at a time."

The next day I woke up and said, "Wow. Are you serious?" I was still seeing white. "You gotta be kidding me. Seriously, this has *got* to be totally temporary. This can't be what I think this is."

Prior to me going blind, I had gone to an optometrist because there had been like a sandy, grainy feeling behind my eyes. It'd seemed like my vision was trying to leave me. The doctors kept telling me there was nothing to worry about though. "Your eyes are normal," they'd told me. "There's nothing wrong with your eyes."

They gave me a pair of glasses just to make me feel comfortable. When my vision went out, at first I thought it might've been those glasses. I said, "Well, maybe they gave me the wrong prescription. I'll just go back to the optometrist and see what's really going on with my eyesight."

I tried to tell my daughter I couldn't see. I couldn't just drive to the doctor's without my vision. I needed her with me to navigate.

At first she was like, "Yeah right, Mommy. You can see."

I said, "No, really. I can't see."

She would not believe me, but we had to go, so she got in the car with me and helped me out. She didn't have a clue on our way there how bad it really was. Everything was ghostly white–I couldn't see any cars in front of me until I was right on their bumper. I couldn't see anything around my peripherals and I couldn't see anything in the mirrors behind me. What little I could see was all white, like I was looking through a thick white sheet and peeking through the fabric. It was very very scary.

Somehow we made it to the optometrist in one piece. The doctor took me back into one of the exam rooms and said, "Okay, let's see what's going on. Read the letters on the wall."

He put up the eye chart and pointed to the one at the very top. I'm looking at the letters and trying to make it out, but I can't see anything but a parallel bar–a parallel bar that's supposed to be the big E. I didn't realize that then, and so as I'm just looking and looking I say, "Well, there's a parallel bar there."

The doctor just looked at my daughter and said, "Who's driving? You or her?"

At that point I figured something was seriously wrong.

Nobody really knew what was going on with me. I went through all this testing and all these exams and the doctors still couldn't figure it out. Everybody understood that I was in school and how important it was that I kept going with it even with all these new challenges. They all knew that this loss was devastating for me, but it was really amazing to see how the doctors, the social workers, my colleagues, my teachers, my friends all came together so I couldn't just give up. Everybody pulled together to do what was necessary for me to continue my education.

My doctor especially helped me continue my education. He was young like me and had just gotten out of college himself. I wanted to get back into college, but I couldn't without any accommodations. The school wasn't going to give me them without an official disability, so I told the doctor, "You know, I want to continue school, but I need some kind of diagnosis in order to qualify for disability and get the accommodations I need to help me stay in school."

He said, "Don't worry about it. This could be a case of Neuromyelitis optica, where you might just have inflammation behind the eyes so your brain is not communicating with them. It might just be a flare up and it might be able to clear up over time. You might be able to see again one day."

So he gave me an official diagnosis, even though he wasn't positive. On paper, I have something called Neuromyelitis optica. It's basically inflammation behind the eyes and a lack of communication with the cord that connects my brain to my eyes. My sight is distorted. I see in like a pixelated view.

Like, have you ever seen *The Matrix*? It's a classic. If you've ever seen it, there's a part toward the end where Neo dies and comes back to life. When he comes back to life you see all these little numbers running down the screen. They're so tiny it's like all pixelated. That's almost how I see.

The doctor didn't know that then. A more accurate diagnosis required tests and exams that I didn't have time for right then. He just looked back at me and said, "Well, I don't know what's going on exactly, but if you are going legally blind, we can get your daughter a permit early so she can drive for you." And then he looked me right in the eyes all serious and said, "You shouldn't try driving. Get home safely and park the car."

I was in denial. We left the doctor's office and my

daughter kinda understood the rules of the road enough to help me navigate, but I didn't let her get a permit because she just wasn't mature enough. She and I just made magic every day together, getting to and from places and whatnot. It was a whole ordeal. She would sit in the passenger seat, I'd sit in the driver's seat, and as I'm driving I'd ask, "Am I in the lane?"

She'd say, "Yeah you're in the lane."

"Can I get over?"

"Sure, you can get over."

"Is the light red, green, or yellow?"

"The light is green, but it's turning yellow."

"When the light turns green, is it okay to make a left?"

"No, there's a car coming."

This is how we drove. It was crazy.

I drove off of her eyesight and her directions. Yes, no, left, right, stay in the lane, make a left, all that. It was really kinda dangerous. I'm blessed we never got in any accidents. But I don't know, I think that maybe because I was a good driver prior to being blind, it worked. I'm still really lucky.

And, oh man, I didn't just need help driving. I relied on my daughter for *everything*.

I went into a deep depression when I lost my vision because I thought my life was over. I thought my career was over. I was a makeup artist, I worked in the spa, I went to school, I was president of FBLA, I was a member of SGA, I had a 3.8 GPA, I was highly active with activities and volunteering, I had a really full plate of things to do. So when my vision went out, it was like my life was over.

It really hurt when I couldn't do makeup anymore. After

I'd lost my vision, I tried to keep it going one last time. One of my regular models was like, "Tonya, I don't trust anyone else to do my makeup. I know you can do it. I'm going to come see you. I don't care if your eyesight is going bad–you can do it."

She was the last face I did. It took me two hours to do what should have taken twenty minutes. I cried after I was done. My daughter assisted me in putting the lashes on, and in the end it still turned out beautiful, but it took way too long. It should have been done quick. The model was like, "Oh, it's so beautiful." But I knew I couldn't go on like that.

I was frustrated. Timing, being a makeup artist, is everything. You have to be able to do your job quickly. Get the models in and out. And now I couldn't do that. So I made a decision. I was like, "This is it. I'm putting my MAC case to the side, I'm getting rid of all my brushes. This is the last face I'll ever do."

I was so hurt. I got to be in such a deep depression that I started being a hermit because I was too scared to go outside by myself. I had to wait until my daughter came home from school. She was scared, too. She tried to organize my things around the house so I knew where everything was, but sometimes I still couldn't find things. I would have to call her while she was in school and I'd say, "Do you know where you put the such in such?" I didn't like doing that. It took away from her lifestyle because she wasn't able to be free. Every time I called, she might've had to rush home to take care of Mom. It was frustrating. It was real real frustrating. I didn't like having to depend on her, and I started thinking I would have to go back home to Chicago to get help from all the family.

One day, my next-door neighbor came over and knocked on my door. Now, my next-door neighbor wasn't just anybody. I lived next door to Kelly Rowland's mom. We were really close–she was like another mother to me. I would always call her Miss Dorris.

She came over and she said, "Are you okay?"

I said, "No, I'm not okay. I gotta go back home, my life is over, my career is over, I can't see, I can't finish school, and I don't know what to do."

And Miss Dorris was so comforting. She told me, "Oh, your life isn't over. You can do all things. Don't worry. You'll be okay. And we're right here with you. You can do this."

Each day I didn't go outside, Miss Dorris would come over and check up on me. She'd come knock on the door. "You wanna come out and get some fresh air? Come on, let's go walk Mocha." Mocha was her little teacup Yorkshire Terrier. Kelly had given her to Miss Dorris and, oh, we would spoil Mocha rotten! We would walk her and once she'd get done walking we'd bring her into the house and wash her in the sink and brush her teeth and put little bows in her hair–she was just like a little person.

Miss Dorris even invited me over for Thanksgiving one time. Kelly and I sat and watched *Devil's Advocate* together–she said it was one of her favorite movies–and Miss Dorris taught me how to make her famous Southern Sweet Tea. It was a family tradition. I am so thankful for Miss Dorris. She really helped me through a difficult time.

Miss Dorris made me get back on track. She made me believe I could still live a life while blind. I decided to go to a bookstore for a magnifier. I was a very avid reader–still am, actually. I would read like six different books at one time so I would have a variety of things to talk about. But when I lost my sight, I had all these books that I couldn't read anymore. That broke my heart. Those books had kept me company.

So I went to the bookstore to get a magnifier. They gave me a seven or eight but I still couldn't see, even with the text magnified that many times. They then referred me to the Center for the Visually Impaired who would possibly have a CCTV for me. A CCTV is like a teleprompter. It's a big-screened computer monitor, like a 27-inch, and you're able to put reading material underneath it. You turn on the actual screen and you can blow the letters all the way up to maybe twenty times the magnification of a normal eye. Usually ten is good enough for me, but I didn't care about the magnification scale. With a CCTV I could read again!

They introduced me to these organizations called National Federation for the Blind and the Department of Human Services. Everybody had heard my story and was so amazed that I was trying. I'll never forget that one of their representatives came to visit me at the school. He said, "You know, you're a unique case."

I was like, "Oh how?"

"Because it appears that you can see, but you really can't. That means it's kinda dangerous for you because others can't tell that you can't see." And then he told me exactly what I did *not* want to hear. "You need to take a cane."

I was like, "Oh no no no no no no no no. This is temporary. I don't need no cane."

"The reason why I say that your life will be a lot easier is because people will know that you're blind," the guy tried.

But I was still like, "Oh no no no no no no no. No no no. I don't want to be vulnerable. I don't want anybody to see me as a walking beacon. No no no. I'm okay. I don't need a cane."

And he said, "Well, you'll have to figure it out on your own time, but I'm letting you know now that it will be safer for you if you take a cane."

I was in denial for about six months. I just didn't want to accept that I needed a cane.

Eventually, I came to accept my blindness, but I wish I didn't have to do it in the way that I did.

I started getting so confident with my driving that one day I was driving by myself, no help. I was doing so good that I even started getting a little aggressive. I probably shouldn't have, but I was. Then all of a sudden this guy cuts me off and blows the light. While he's cutting me off, I try to navigate between two lanes to get out of his way, but there's a black Mercedes Benz sitting right in front of me. I didn't see it. It was black like the road so I couldn't see it.

I hit it.

Those things are like tanks. It didn't take too much damage, but the whole trunk popped off and a baby seat flew out onto the hood of my car. I think it was from the trunk, but I'm not sure. I didn't know where it was from at the time. As soon as I saw that car seat, I just went into shock. I thought a baby might've been in it. I was like, "Oh my God! Oh my God! I just killed a baby, I just killed a baby. Oh my God!" I think I'm a very loving and caring person, so any harm of life is devastating to me, especially a baby. I couldn't handle it.

The fire department got there and the police got there and it turned out that everything was okay. Luckily, there was no baby in the car seat. But I was still freaking out. The lady who was in the Mercedes was like, "Oh, you don't have to worry. Accidents happen. It's okay. I just dropped off my granddaughter."

But while I'm freaking out and crying and being absolutely devastated, nobody knew *why* I was acting like that. Why I was in shock. It looks like I can see, remember? They didn't know I was blind. I was in shock because it was irresponsible for me to be driving, and I was just then really realizing how irresponsible it was. I could've killed a baby. It was like a total mind job for me. I was freaking out–so much so that I could feel chills going all the way down my legs. Cold chills. It felt terrible.

The paramedics were like, "Are you sure *you* don't need to go to the hospital? You sure that you're all right?"

I was the one who hit the lady, but *she* was more concerned about *me*. I was more concerned about the whole situation and wishing it'd never happened.

Now here's the crazy thing. My mother had come down from Minnesota two weeks before that accident. When she found out I was driving she was like, "Okay, time to pick it up. We're going home."

Mona Sha'e didn't want to go. She was like, "No, Mommy. We can handle it, we can handle it."

And then the randomest thing happened! I was going through a lot of testing because they were trying to figure out what was wrong with me (still) and I just happened to be at the doctor's office for a CAT scan. There was this lady waiting there who was also getting a CAT scan. She just turned and started talking with us. I don't know how she knew I was blind too, because I didn't have a cane. I guess we just kinda recognized each other? Felt it on some other level. I don't know. All I know is that we ran into this lady who was visually impaired and she told my mom, "Oh, your daughter will be just fine. We've got a great community here and she can adjust. She'll be fine. Let her figure her way out. Don't take her independence away."

My mom said, "Well, do you know that she *drives* and my *granddaughter* is navigating? Now how can I get her to stop driving?"

The lady just said, "Look. Something's gonna happen where she's gonna have to figure it out and she's gonna eventually have to put it down. Hopefully she won't hurt nobody, but you got to let her figure that out for herself because the last thing a person wants to let go of is driving. That's part of their independence."

And lo and behold, two weeks later I get in that accident.

I had just bought me a brand new Ford Taurus show performance vehicle too. It had a V8 engine, duel over exhaust, duel overhead cam, all the bells and whistles. Yeah, I loved my cars. I really did. I babied my cars so it was a beaut. We called her Strawberry.

But then when I hit the car and the whole trunk popped off I was like, "Okay that's it. I'm not driving no more. That's *it*...Unless I have to go to the grocery store."

No seriously! The grocery store was right down the street. Literally. Like you had Publix right there and Garden of Eden right next to it and so the grocery stores were literally right down the street. Sha'e and I could hop in the car and go get our groceries and come back right quick. I guess it took me a little longer to give that up, but we had to eat! Outside of going to the store, I didn't drive anywhere else.

Losing my vision was a total lifestyle change for me. I had to start doing things differently, I had to start asking for help, I had to start learning how to use the bus, I had to start my life all over again. With all the things that were different, though, one thing stayed the same: I made sure that no matter what, I would keep on going to college until I finished my degree.

4 | Back to Business School

I never stopped going to school. I couldn't afford to stop going because once I lost my vision, I couldn't work anymore. I had to rely on my student loans to support me and my daughter. School became my full time job after blindness.

At first, I had to start taking public transportation and cabs and whatnot, and because I wouldn't take a cane, I would run across the street like I was playing *Frogger*. I'd just run across the street, crossing my fingers and hoping I wouldn't get hit. I wasn't trained at the time. I'd just sprint across saying, "Don't hit me don't hit me don't hit me don't hit me–okay I made it!" You know how dangerous that is? Pretty dangerous. And Buckhead had some very busy streets.

Finally one day Miss Dorris said, "Tonya, if you've got to go to school, I'll take you in the morning and drop you off. You just cross the street at the light where everybody else does and get in there safely. I don't want you running across the streets like that." And so every morning Miss Dorris would come and get me, and then she'd drive me and drop me off at school, and all I would have to do was catch a cab back home. We did that every day.

It was really interesting because I was the first person who was blind at my school. They didn't really know how to deal with it. It was kinda hurtful for me because they really didn't want to invest because they felt they had to invest a lot. For them, it was always, "Well, how much money?" I was president of FBLA, liaison to the AMBCC, a member of SGA, had a really good GPA, and they didn't want to invest in me. They didn't want to invest in me as a person with a visual impairment.

For each accommodation, it was pretty much all the same: "All this extra stuff? I don't know. I don't think we wanna put a computer over here. Well how much is that gonna cost?" It was hurtful.

Luckily, the Department of Human Services and the National Federation for the Blind decided to invest in me. They wanted to help me continue on with my life.

The Department of Human Services introduced me to a program called Kurzweil 3000. It's a text-to-speech program for the blind and dyslexic so they can read on their computer. DHS also put zoom text on their computer for me. They also gave me that CCTV, too, when I was first starting to take back my life. It took a while for me to accept audiobooks, so I needed the CCTV. I like to hold a book, not just listen to it. When they tried to get me to read audiobooks, I was like, "No! That's cheating!" Now I listen to them, though.

I met two very important people in my life from National Federation for the Blind: Anil Lewis and Garrett Scott. They were always so inspiring to me because they pushed me to be the best version of me I could be with this new blindness. They always told me, "Blindness is not a disability. It's a characteristic!"

They came and sat down with me to give me the same spiel about getting a cane, too. "It doesn't appear to everyone else that you can't see, but you can't," they'd told me. "You need to carry a cane. It's for your own safety. If you carry a cane, other people know that you can't see. So if you bump into somebody they won't be upset. Or if you're crossing the street and a car thinks that you really can see, they might hit you. Or if you're walking down the street and there's an open manhole that you don't see, you might fall in it." And then they said, "You won't have to explain to people over and over that you're visually impaired."

That was a problem I was noticing as I was getting out more. I would go places, like a restaurant for example, and I would go try to order something to eat. I'd be like, "What do you guys have?"

"Can't you read that sign right there?"

And then I'd get frustrated. "I'm legally blind."

"Oh, oh, oh, I'm sorry."

It was a problem. I might ask someone, "What time is it?"

They'd be like, "Don't you see the clock? You can't tell time?"

Or they would think that you're illiterate because you couldn't read. You know, all those things. I started seeing all those different troubles and I was frustrated, but I still didn't want to be carrying a cane. I just refused to carry one. I was still in denial, thinking my vision would come back at any point. I just kept dealing with all those intricacies and I thought that if I carried a cane I would be a walking target. I thought it'd be dangerous for me to be going around letting everyone know how vulnerable I was. In actuality, though, it was more dangerous that I wasn't carrying one.

I had to work even harder in school, too. Everyone was like, "Why don't you just go to one of those schools for blind people?"

I just told them, "Nah, I want to finish my degree."

What really stuck out to me about continuing my education after losing my vision was that I had to work three times as hard to keep up with my fellow students. I wasn't going to work anymore, so I had nothing but time on my hands (and I had to depend on student loans, which I hadn't had to before). What occupied my time was studying and keeping my grades up so I could continue to get those loans and grants and scholarships to get through school. The cost of it was challenging since I didn't have a job to pay for it.

But the people really received me and my daughter well. My counselors, my teachers, Mr. Breelin, Dr. Laurent, all of them. I had a strong support system and my family wasn't even around, which was amazing.

The Department of Human Services was especially generous. For Christmas that year, they gave me like a 27-inch screen computer, a portable CCTV, a recorder, Kurzweil 3000, ZoomText, they even gave me a dolly to carry all my equipment on. Oh, it was crazy! And they didn't just get me equipment. They gave me some gifts, too, like my favorite movie, *Falling Down*, and a cute gray sweater. They even gave my daughter some gifts. She got an mp3 player and some other things, too.

They gave me and my daughter a Christmas. It was like we didn't even miss a beat. Nobody would allow us to. Everyone just wanted us to keep on keeping on and nobody would let me give up. All that love was really crazy.

Things started really looking up for me. But, of course, then things just didn't. There was one situation at Herzing that really didn't go well.

I was already disgruntled with my school, but then I had this one professor. You know how you have some teachers who are good teachers and some teachers who aren't good teachers but they're good at their profession? I had one like that. It was an accounting class and he was supposedly a top-notch accountant. He didn't know how to teach though! He would try to explain things to us and then when we'd all just look at him, not understanding, he'd say, "Okay, well, never mind. Here's the answer."

And, by now I'm sure you know how I am, so I was like, "Oh no, that's not acceptable. We gotta learn how to do it ourselves!"

I'm a student who learns by asking questions. I wanted to make sure I knew the processes and not just the answers. I spoke up a lot in that class and I don't think he liked that very much. I don't think he liked me very much.

I was having a hard time being on time for class because

I'd still been trying to adjust to being blind–finding things, organizing, getting to school, all that. It's really a challenge being physically challenged. You've got to go through so much preparation just to do anything. The simplest of things. And so when I would arrive late, that professor would give me a whole different curriculum from everybody else and it would be much more difficult too. He'd sit me in the back of the class where I couldn't see and then he would give me these outrageous equations to figure out. It was awful!

When course evaluations came around, I typed up a nice long letter about how he wasn't a good professor. I was all, "We're supposed to be representations of the school once we graduate and if we can't get out there and do things in the real world, if we can't operate as accountants, then how does that look for Herzing? This is unacceptable for him to just give us answers without explanations and blah blah blah blah." Yeah, I was definitely in FBLA mode!

He knew exactly who sent the response even though I didn't put my name on it. Who else could it have been? He was really out for me after that. I had to get one of my accounting mentors to tutor me and I paid him $50 per tutoring session to get me through the class.

I was doing okay after that. Around this time, the National Federation for the Blind was going to offer me a scholarship. They were like, "Hey, Tonya. You've got a good GPA, and if you keep it up, we'll get you a scholarship to get you through school." All of this was working in my favor, and it was a nice pick-me-up during my class with that professor.

Unfortunately, something happened.

My daughter was in the wrong place at the wrong time. She got caught up in some trouble and I couldn't get to her fast enough. My daughter had problems with other children at school and an emergency had occurred with her where I had to drop everything to tend to her. I had to go before a judge and everything. I told the judge, "My daughter has never been in trouble before. She was in the wrong place at the wrong time. I just became blind and there might be a lot of factors in this equation." The court case took a long time.

Meanwhile, Herzing gave me like thirty to ninety days to make up my finals because of that incident. I was so busy with my daughter that I didn't finish them until right at the deadline. I sent in those finals at midnight the day they were due, but for some reason the email never went through. All of the final tests that I took–the tests that I know I could've gotten A's on–were graded as F's. My professor, the one who didn't like me, wouldn't give me any leeway.

And the school stood behind his decision.

I was so hurt and heartbroken. Those F's really infected my GPA. Plus, the case wasn't looking good, so I ended up telling the judge, "Well, I'll go back home and I'll have my family help me raise my daughter. I need the help. I'm blind."

This was when I finally realized that my eyesight wasn't coming back.

The judge said that that would be okay, so I moved back home to Minnesota with my daughter. My mother is from Minnesota, and a lot of my family is there, but I still had to leave the support system I'd built in Atlanta. All of my friends. Everyone was like, "Are you serious? You're leaving?"

I told them, "Yeah, I gotta do what I need to do for my daughter."

It was almost funny, because the school kinda flipped their perspective on me and begged me to stay. I was like, "No. If you guys did this to me because you didn't want to accommodate me and my disability, you'll do it again. If I allow you to get away with this, you'll just do it again. I gotta go."

And so I uprooted myself and left the whole support system that I'd built, all of my friends who were more like family, and I went back to Minnesota. I went back to get help.

And maybe I'd finally get a cane, too.

5 | BLIND, Inc.

When I first got to Minneapolis, Minnesota, I went through a lot of grief. I'd lost my vision and I was finally coming to terms with that fact. I was kinda forced to accept it. There was no other reason for me going home. I needed help to manage my blindness. I would cry all the time, depressed.

But I always tried to lift myself up and keep moving. That was important. One thing I've noticed through this whole journey is how some people are hurt emotionally by something happening to them physically. They may be so bitter and mean, but they're like that because they're hurt, and when you're really angry like that, you take it out on people. You push people away who want to help you, even though you shouldn't. It's no good to be negative.

I've always tried to have a level of gratitude because people have always been very warm and welcoming and helpful toward me. They don't have to either. That's their prerogative.

So I'm even more grateful for the people who have helped me along the way. I'm grateful that they are there, and that they are genuine, and that they really want to help. I'm a very independent person, but whenever someone offers their help, I'm so grateful. One way or another, I find my way through the maze of everything I'm going through, and when I have to do things on my own, a lot of people are like, "How'd you do that?"

I always tell them, "Well, I just told myself that I'm going to try it and if it don't work, oh well."

That's my attitude. You've gotta stay positive. You've gotta keep moving.

This bout of depression was over quicker than the first time I dealt with depression back in Atlanta. I was lucky because once I moved to Minneapolis, I had a direction to go in. Back in Georgia when I was getting everything ready for the move, I told Anil and Garrett from the National Federation for the Blind that I was leaving. They asked me where I was going, and when I said I was going to Minnesota they told me, "Oh, look up BLIND, Inc. It's the best training facility for the visually impaired in the country. Part of the NFB."

BLIND, Inc. was in this building called the Pillsbury Mansion. You know the Pillsbury Dough Boy, the one that giggles when you poke his tummy? Their family donated the Pillsbury Mansion to BLIND, Inc.

They had some awesome programs, and it looked really nice, so I decided to go.

The program was a little scary at first, though. You would have to leave home and they would put you in your own apartment. You couldn't see your family for the first sixty days. I was like, "What do you mean I can't see my family?" The whole point of the program was to become independent, though, so they wanted to get you away from being attached to someone. Away from being dependent on someone else.

And so, of course, the first thing I had to do was get a cane.

It wasn't as terrible as I thought it was, though. When I took a cane, it was like a whole new world of freedom had opened up for me. I didn't have to wait for somebody to take me somewhere or need somebody to hold my hand to guide me or have somebody to tell me what's there and what's not. I was able to maneuver on my own with no problem.

From the apartment, we would have to catch the bus every morning to get to Pillsbury Mansion. I'd do this just visually impaired—I can kinda see in like a pixelated view, remember?—but as soon as we hit the steps of the Pillsbury Mansion, we put on sleep shades. Everyone puts on sleep shades so we're all at the same level of blindness. You can't see *a thing*. No one can see anything but total darkness while training at BLIND, Inc.

Then once you've got your shades on, it's time for classes. Oh, there were some *amazing* instructors. It was ridiculous. They were like superheroes. There's someone who teaches life skills, someone who teaches braille, someone who teaches technology, and then someone who teaches you how to travel.

Emily taught braille and she was a really sweet lady. Learning braille with her was interesting. We got to learn how to use the stencil, which was really *really* interesting. You use it if you need to take notes. Normally if you can see, to take notes you grab a piece of paper and you just write down the note real quick. Well, a blind person can't write it down on a piece of paper because they can't see it. So they have the stencil. It's like a metal contraption where you open it up and close it on top of the paper. Then you pull it down, pull it closed, and you have this punch that's almost like an ice pick. And then you just punch in each stencil, making holes through the paper so when you go over it and take the stencil out, you can feel those bumps.

There was also this technology called BrailleNote. It's like a little device where you can type your braille and the braille comes up on like a rubber pad. Real high-tech, right?

There's also a typewriter and a few other machines that help with braille, but before you get into all these complicated things, you have to start out with that stencil. You have to learn your ABC's, your one-two-three's, and then you move your way up from there.

In technology, we learned how to work with assisted technology such as JAWS (Job Access With Speech). JAWS is like a text to speech reader for your computer that reads the words right on the screen. There were some people who could read up to almost a hundred and fifty words a minute! I mean, they would be listening, but that's still really fast. To me, JAWS would just be like, "dadadadadada." Just really really fast, like a blur. The average person can't read that fast, hearing-wise.

I don't read that fast either. If I'm telling you the truth, I'm just too intimidated. I can't do that. I think I'm more of a visual person. Kinda ironic, huh? Everyone was like, "Tonya, you wanna try it out?"

"I'm reading six words a minute," I'd say. "Maybe ten. But I'm okay."

I'm a ZoomText person. I like to zoom it up real big because I'm so nosy. I'm scared that if I'm listening, I'm going to miss out on something.

Or maybe I'm just stubborn. Like when I didn't want the cane. Who knows?

So yeah, technology class was cool, learning braille was fun, but those classes were nowhere near as awesome as the other two.

Life Skills especially was great. There was another Emily at BLIND, Inc. and she taught that one. She'd have us do some of the most amazing stuff. She would always say, "You don't stop doing things. You just do things differently."

And it was true! We'd learn how to change light bulbs and how to pour a glass of water and how to organize our clothes and even how to make bookshelves and desks and chairs in woodshop! We learned all sorts of stuff that you do at home—stuff you probably don't think twice about if you can see, huh? It was amazing.

So say I wanted to pour me some juice or a glass of water. How would I know when to stop pouring so the cup doesn't overflow? Well, Emily taught us to hold our thumb right at the edge of the glass, about an inch away from the top. That way, as you're pouring, you stop when you feel the liquid. You have successfully filled the glass.

Or maybe I wanted to get dressed, but how do I know if my outfit matches if I can't see the colors? Well, we learned how to organize our clothes. They have this machine that scans your clothes and tells you the color. It's a meter that you can use to sort by color, and it can tell you the colors, like red, green, blue, yellow, all the basic colors. But some are so sophisticated! They'll be like turquoise, light blue, pink purple, aqua blue! And then I'd have everything sorted by type, too. I wore suits all the time, so I'd have all my suits in one section. Then in another, I'd have my shirts. I'd have my slacks, my dresses, my casual clothes, everything organized as the outfits I wanted to wear, in the colors I wanted to wear. I just grab the outfit and go. I must have looked so stylish because people were always like, "You pick out your own clothes?"

I'd just tell them, "I sure do."

Or maybe I wanted to get some cooking done. How do I know what ingredients I have and how much I need and all the little things that you wouldn't normally think about if you can see? Well, the stove would be marked so you could know where the buttons and dials were and whatnot. The instructors would put the food out for you so you didn't have to go digging for anything in the fridge or the cabinets. And then we'd cook! We're using butcher knives and everything to cut up our food, putting our food right on the stove, we're doing everything just like anybody who could see would do. The only difference is they showed us safety mechanisms to protect us from intense heat and how to set our timers correctly and how to fill that measuring cup up to the right level and all that. Cooking was always my favorite lesson in Life Skills.

And when you're finished cooking, you've got to clean up your mess, right? But how do you know what's dirty and what's not? With dishes, you could hand wash them but you won't know how clean it is–you can't see any leftover grime. That's why a dishwasher is very important to a blind person. You can prewash and then throw it in the dishwasher and then you *know* it's clean. Or with cleaning the countertop and other surfaces, you just run your hand over it. You feel the grain and grit and you wipe it down right there. When you sweep the floor, you do a routine where you sweep around all the cracks and crevices along the walls and make your way toward the middle of the floor and that's it. Whether there's trash there or not, you still sweep it. That way, you know everything's been swept. It's important to stay organized like that and have your routines down solid. When you're someone who is visually impaired, you have to remember that you can still live independently–you just have to know your environment and how everything is organized.

What it all boils down to is organization. Everything about being visually impaired and living on your own is about organization. If you're not organized, you lose time, and that's time you can't get back. Everything has its designated place. Your plates are here, your utensils are there–*everything has a place*. I'm so organized that when I'm around other people they think I'm anal. I'm not though. I *need* to be organized, because if I'm not, my whole way of life gets thrown out of whack. Whenever someone comes over, I'm always like, "Don't touch anything! If you touch something or move something, then I have to figure out what you did with it."

Life Skills taught me so much, but it was the travel class that really let my independence flourish.

We had this travel instructor whose name was Zach. And you could never forget Zach. Zach was like a real superhero. He was Superman! You never really knew the degree of a person's blindness, and with Zach, it was like he wasn't even blind. He would jump on the staircase's banister and slide right on down. Then he'd jump off and tap the floor with his cane. "Let's rock and roll!"

Everybody would just laugh whenever Zach did this. The first time I met him I was like, "Zach, how blind are you really?"

And he says, "Well, that's for me to know and for you to find out."

But he *was* blind. I just thought this dude was absolutely amazing! He taught us how to get around and how to use our canes. You've got to tap your way up the stairs. You've got to tap your way to the bus stop. You've got to tap your way to the kitchen. You've got to tap your way everywhere. You've got to use your cane.

Zach taught us how to rely on our other senses to get around. He was the one who taught me how to really listen for cars. He'd take us out, make us cross the street–right in the middle of it, too, no crosswalks or anything–and we'd have to listen to hear if any cars were coming or not. And if you don't hear any cars, you listen for anything else that might be dangerous. If nothing's there, you feel the curb with your cane, you step down, you make sure there aren't any parked cars around or parked motorcycles or other vehicles or whatever, and then you cross. You have to make sure you're walking in a straight line, too, because you don't want to be walking on an angle. You might just keep walking down the street if your angle is off!

But people don't just cross streets to cross streets. You've got places to be! So how do we know when we get somewhere we want to go if we can't see what's around us? We have to memorize streets, and Zach taught us the secret to it: you count them.

For example, you're on 29th Avenue and you want to go to Hennepin Avenue. Those two are cross streets so it's just a straight shot down 29th. But what's the next street over. Is it Nicollet? Or is it something else? You would have to count the streets. And as you're walking, you'd be like, "Okay, that's one block. That's two blocks." You can tell when you've gone a block, too, because the street drops. There's the curb. So how many blocks are you counting? How many blocks did you go this way? Are you going north, south, east, or west? What streets are going this way and what streets are going that way? Just walking a few blocks is a whole ordeal when you're visually impaired.

Sometimes we had tests. They'd take us to a random spot in the middle of the city and have us put our blindfolds on and we'd have to get back to the mansion or some other predetermined spot all on our own. No help whatsoever. The teacher is always there–even when you think he's not–to make sure you don't hurt yourself, but he'd never help you or give you directions. You're just sitting there by yourself, clicking and clicking and clicking and clicking. It can be real frustrating. You know someone's there, but you also know that they're not going to help you one bit. So all of your disappointed groans and personal curse words and all that, they're there to hear it. You're just clicking around, getting more and more irritated, and they're just watching you. I bet it was probably funny for them sometimes.

You could get lost in a parking lot for hours, just trying to figure your way out. Those exercises were to help you learn the difference in how each tap of the cane sounds and feels. What a tap on the sidewalk sounds like. What a crack in the pavement feels like. You should be able to tell if there's grass over here, or if there's a curb ahead that you're about to step down from, or if you're coming to a corner or door before you walk into it–you should be able to tell what everything is, or at least have some educated guess. You keep your cane three feet in front of you so you won't trip and fall. You're supposed to feel with your cane, almost like the cane is part of you. It's an extension of you. You're tapping, you're feeling vibrations, you're listening. You're doing all of this because you can't see.

It's all superhuman stuff, I'm telling you! We would take field trips sometimes to different National Federation of the Blind conventions and meet these people who not only had to deal with their physical challenges, but also had amazing professional careers. They were completely independent and it was so encouraging to see! When I saw how amazing these people were, these teachers who were just as blind as we were, I said, "There ain't nothing I can't do if they can do it. These are superheroes right here!" They were all so inspiring, and they gave me a new, more positive outlook on my life.

See, the thing is, when you become visually impaired, it's like a whole 'nother world that's actually kind of beautiful. I know that sounds crazy, but it's like reading a book. You're hearing how everything is being described and you make a picture in your mind. In your mind you can be more creative, instead of just taking what you see at face value. You can enjoy things more because you get to picture what you want to picture. I mean, at one point in time I got so comfortable with being visually impaired that I was like, "I'm glad there are some things I just can't see." I would make that joke sometimes. These people at BLIND, Inc. taught me that it was okay to be okay with my visual impairment. It was just another part of me. I didn't have to be reduced to being "the blind person". Being blind is just a small part of who I am as a person. I can do anything a seeing person can do, and maybe even more.

Later on in life (and in this book), I was really really sick. I was so sick that I was bedridden at my mom's apartment. I couldn't feed myself, I couldn't move around the apartment, I couldn't do anything on my own. I was literally drinking everything through a straw. A friend came to visit me one day, and after chatting and whatnot, he was like, "Man, I need something to drink."

Now, I didn't know the house. I'd never been there before being released from the hospital, and I couldn't see any of the rooms inside. But I knew where everything was. I was like, "Just go in the kitchen, there to your right, and look in the cupboard over the sink. That's where the glasses are."

Or he'd say, "Oh, I need some forks."

And I'd tell him, "If you go in that drawer across the way, under the microwave, you should find some utensils there."

It wasn't just the kitchen either. I knew where everything

was in the house.

"I need a towel to wash my hands."

"Oh, if you go to that second door in the hallway, probably on the third shelf, that's where the towels will be."

My friend was amazed. He was like, "Tonya. It absolutely amazes me that you are bedridden but know every inch of this house. You can tell me where everything is just using your other senses."

I didn't realize it when I was helping him out, but I knew everything from what I would hear every day when my mother moved around. I heard everything, and because I had my training from BLIND, Inc. I knew what each sound meant. I could rely on those other senses. It was really something special, even after all the years that had passed since my training.

To graduate from the program, you had to take one of those tests. They would drop you off in the middle of the city and you had to find your way back to the Pillsbury mansion within two hours. I never got to take the test, never got to officially graduate, because I left the program before that could happen. I'm sure I could have aced that test, though.

The training I received from BLIND, Inc. was phenomenal. If I hadn't gone, I don't think I'd have been able to accomplish what I've done since. To this day I'm using techniques I learned while there.

I owe a lot to BLIND, Inc.

6 | Super Student

BLIND, Inc. gave me a lot of independence, so much so that I decided to go back to college.

I went to Metropolitan State University because they had this program called "First College". It's still there today, it's just called "The College of Individual Studies" now. With First College, you could write your own degree. But it's not as simple as it sounds. You have to do a few training classes first. You have to go through a critical thinking class, and after that you do a self-development class, and then you take a class on how to write your own degree plan. Finally you have to take a class that shows you how to convert the college education and life experiences that you already have and turn them into credits. Easy peasy, right? Not.

Well, when I heard of it, I didn't care about all that work. I was just like, "What? Oh yeah, let me make a degree for entrepreneurship."

I came up with a Bachelor's in Entrepreneurship because I had studied business administration and accounting at Herzing and I had so many years in already that I didn't want to lose my credit hours. So I converted those hours and I changed the degree from business management to entrepreneurship. I wanted to open my own spa resort one day and be an entrepreneur, so why not study it?

Even with all those classes you had to take beforehand that helped you learn how to make a degree plan, it's still much harder to write your own versus having one premade. But I did it. You would come up with a degree, pick out the classes you thought would compliment it, get the plan approved by the department head, and then if you wanted to do an independent study instead of an individual class, you'd have to get those approved too.

You can pick whatever classes you want—at any college you want, too, since you can convert life experience and college courses that were outside Metro State—but you have to research them first to see how you can get them to fit. Like, for example, I studied Improvisational Jazz at Walker West Academy. I love jazz and put the class into my degree plan just because I really like jazz. But I had to explain it in terms of my program. I said that I felt like I needed to use both sides of my brain in order to learn more efficiently and then explained how music helps do that. It lowers stress and encourages creativity and all that. Really, though, I just wanted to learn how to play by ear. I've played the flute since the second grade, but up until I lost my vision, I was *reading* sheet music. I couldn't read music like that anymore, and I didn't know how to play without it, so I wanted to learn how.

Now, with those classes, I ended up breaking the First College mold. They even changed the program rules because of me. Reason being I wrote my Master's into my undergrad and earned a Master's degree in Nonprofit Organizational Management. We technically weren't supposed to do that.

Here's how I did it.

I got there and said, "Huh. I can really get my money's worth out of this. What if I wrote my Master's into my Undergrad?" So I asked and one of the counselors for the program–not my actual counselor, because she was out on sabbatical at the time–was real adamant. "Oh no no no no," she told me. "You can't do that. You have to stay in the requirements of undergrad. No no no no."

She was a real mean lady. I just said, "Okay".

But knowing me, I didn't stop there. I read the descriptions for the classes I really wanted to take and at the bottom of each one it said, *Requirement: Bachelor's degree or permission from each professor.*

Yeah. I bet you can tell what I did next. Brilliant me would go and ask each individual professor if could I take their class to get my Master's into my degree plan. I'd tell them that I was a part of First College and I'd show them my background and I'd do everything I could to get them to give me the okay. And each one did. I would have to get each professor of each Master's class to sign off for me to take the class each semester. I didn't *have* to go through that whole process if I would have just done a regular undergrad, but going the normal route didn't make sense when I could've saved the time and money with this First College program. So I went around that counselor's back and wrote my Master's degree into my undergrad degree.

I started going to Metro State at the same time I was going to BLIND, Inc. I went simultaneously and I was the only person who did both. I would have to leave BLIND, Inc. halfway through the day to go to my college classes, and it wasn't a problem at first. I was doing both for a good six to eight months. But I guess what happened was my going back and forth encouraged other students to do the same thing. My colleagues wanted to go back to school too. BLIND, Inc. didn't like that. They wanted me to choose between the program and the college. BLIND, Inc. was like, "You have to go to this program full time. It's either school or here."

I was like, "Well, I came here so I could finish school, so I think I'd better take school."

It was a bittersweet departure. I had to leave in December, right around Christmastime. I had to pack up my BLIND, Inc. apartment in like forty-eight hours all by myself. It was a lot. When I was finally done and went home to my mommy, my knee was hurting really really bad. I didn't really think nothing of it. I just decided to take it easy for the rest of the day.

The very next day, I went to visit my cousin in Wisconsin for Christmas and New Year's. I got there, though, and I started having trouble breathing. When I lay down to go to sleep, it would hurt to breathe. I could feel my lungs being constricted each time I took a breath. I didn't know what was going on. I mean, I was crying because I could barely breathe.

Finally my cousin just told me, "Go to the emergency

room!" I wasn't thinking about being sick. I was like the bill of health–minus my vision, of course. Why would I go to the emergency room if I wasn't sick? Lo and behold, I ended up in the emergency room anyway.

When I got there, they were trying to figure out what was going on with me. They couldn't figure it out, and they didn't get any leads until they put me in for a CAT scan. I couldn't lie down flat, though. I couldn't breathe that way. The doctor came back to me after that and looked me in the eyes and started crying. It wasn't much, just a few tears were rolling, but he said, "You're too young for this. If you didn't come any sooner, you probably wouldn't have made it. You've got blood clots in your lungs."

The blood clot had traveled from my knee and all the way up to my lungs. I had injured my knee three days prior to my departure from BLIND, Inc. while catching the bus to school, standing up on my legs for forty-eight hours without really taking any time to sit and rest while I was doing a bunch of packing after that injury had helped contribute to the blood clot. I had overworked myself.

I had to be admitted. I couldn't breathe and that clot could have stopped my heart, or worse, it could have gone to my brain, giving me an aneurism and possibly killing me. It was life-threatening and so I had to stay. I think all of the staff and everyone there probably sympathized with me because I had to be in the hospital for both Christmas and New Year's. They were awesome. They made it feel like I wasn't even in a hospital. It felt really nice.

I was there for two weeks. They still didn't really want to

let me go home because they were trying to balance out my blood clots and they had me on medication and all that. But I had to get back to school. The spring semester was starting soon and I wanted to be there. I didn't care about the danger. If I died trying to learn, that's what I would do. I wasn't going to give up.

When I got home, everyone wasn't so sure about my decision to return to school. My mom was like, "Tonya, are you really okay?" The school was like, "Are you sure you're not too sick?" Everyone! I had to explain myself over and over. "Look," I'd tell someone whenever they asked. "I'm not going to stay sitting around. If I go out, I go out my way. I want to learn!" So, stubborn me, I stayed at Metropolitan State University.

I went right back to school when the Spring semester started. I was really weak, but I still went. Because of the blood clots and the dangers of them possibly traveling to my lungs or my heart or my brain, I would have to go get my blood drawn two to three times a week. They would test my blood levels because I was taking Heparin, which shares its active ingredient with rat poison. They use rat poisoning to thin the rat's blood to kill them, so the same ingredient is in some medications. If your blood gets too thin, you can bleed to death, but if your blood is too thick then you've got to be careful about getting more clots. It was very scary, pretty life-threatening, but I wasn't going to let it stop me from my education.

I went to school full-time, no jobs or anything to keep me away from my studies. Metro State was more accommodating for me and my disability than Herzing was, too. I got my classes approved like three weeks before the course catalog opened to everybody else because I had to purchase my books from the bookstore and then we would have to send my books out to Recording for the Blind & Dyslexic (now named Learning Ally). They would record audio formats of my books and send them back on a jump drive so I could put it on my computer to listen to. Since I'd already had my classes picked weeks in advance, I'd have it in time for class. If I didn't get that accommodation, I would have received my audiobooks in the middle of class. I would already be behind.

There were other accommodations too, and thanks to my training from BLIND, Inc. and all that I was now able to do on my own, some of my able-bodied classmates just didn't get it. They'd be like, "Why are you carrying a cane?"

I'd tell them, "Because I'm visually impaired."

It took them awhile to realize that because I took a totally different approach to my visual impairment. Instead of wearing the big blue blockers that most blind people wear, I wore Coco Chanel sunglasses. I needed my bling. And I wore them every day, all day long–it didn't matter where I was. I'd wear them at night, indoors, during class. People would ask me, "Who do you think you are? A superstar?"

And I was used to it. I'd just explain to them, "No, my eyes actually have a sensitivity to light, but I don't want you to feel sorry for me and say, 'Oh, you poor baby.' So I wear these nice Coco Chanel glasses."

I didn't want anybody feeling bad for me. I just kinda owned my blindness and made it me. I think BLIND, Inc. gave me that independence, and it helped me realize I could live on my own and do whatever I set my mind to.

Living on my own was really something special, especially with my First College degree plan. Home was like my haven now that I had the training to be independent. I could do anything I wanted. I would listen to music, I would play my flute, I'd watch the birds that would come chirp by my window, I'd hop on my elliptical machine, I'd cook, I'd write, I'd just take time to relax during all the schoolwork. That's what I think is important about learning–or at least that's how it worked for me. I couldn't just grill grill grill grill with no enjoyment, no fun. I'd work and then I'd take a break. And the work wasn't super boring, either, which really helped. It was more a learning experience versus a "I gotta get this degree so I can go earn some money" kind of thing. It was actually something I wanted to do, so that made the learning experience more enjoyable. That's what First College was supposed to be about.

With me being independent and really liking First College, naturally my next step was getting involved in a bunch of extracurriculars again. First I joined the Student Senate. I'd already been a part of the Student Government Association at Herzing and I was a little disgruntled by how they didn't take care of me back in Georgia. So when I went to Metro they kept approaching me and asking, "Hey, you wanna join Student Senate?" I was always like, "No." I didn't want to get sucked back into politics.

But they kept asking and asking, just like at Herzing, and finally someone came to me–I think it might've been the president or the vice president of Student Senate, but I'm not sure–and they made me feel really really guilty for not being a part of the senate. They told me, "You know, Tonya, we're here to represent the student body of Metro State. And we don't have anyone who's physically challenged. We need a voice for those who have challenges. Would you deprive your fellow students of that right? You could be the voice for them."

They'd broken me down. I was like, "Okay. You got me. Let's do this."

So, reluctantly, I joined the student senate.

Around that time, Obama was running for president. We had a big *Get Out The Vote* campaign that was really huge on our campus. We set up booths, we had a couple of days where people could come to the campus to vote, we gave out information on the candidates who were running at the time, we hosted get-togethers at the library where everybody could come and watch the debates on these big screen TVs we had, we were all in. That *Get Out The Vote* campaign was just like its own total culture outside of being a student. If I wasn't doing my schoolwork or if I wasn't in class, I was working with the student senate for *Get Out The Vote*. When we hosted that initiative, we also would go on trips to different schools. It was on one of these trips that I learned about MnSCU.

MnSCU is the Minnesota State Colleges and Universities system. What they do is write policies and plans and procedures for schools throughout the state. They govern tuition costs, insurance policies, stuff like that. At the time, they didn't have anyone representing the disabled population, so, of course, I was recruited to join.

Being a part of MnSCU was pretty cool because it was like all these different colleges from around the state of Minnesota and we'd go and spend all day in all these different meetings and conventions. There'd be different topics at each one, like we'd discuss school technology at one or university curriculum at another. There was always something different to talk about with MnSCU.

We would visit different colleges as a part of that program and find out what they needed to do to improve their experience in college. We'd see if they needed to change a school policy or if we could help out with their health insurance, since there was a big thing about students not being able to stay on their parents' insurance at the time. We actually had a lot to do with that movement. We lobbied, going all the way to Washington to do it. I, myself, didn't get to go to Washington, but some of my MnSCU team went to get certain initiatives passed. Basically we just travelled all over Minnesota writing policies and programs to enhance college students' lives. It was awesome.

I didn't just travel as a part of MnSCU though. I wrote a lot of travel into my degree plan as a life experience program with a spa in Dilworth, North Carolina. Dilworth is a real affluent neighborhood in Charlotte where the houses all look the same and everybody's driving a Mercedes Benz and everything. It was real nice. But the reason I was there was to help build the team for a spa called Elite Experience.

My cousin who I had visited in Wisconsin that winter eventually relocated to North Carolina. She's always had a surplus of money and had decided she wanted to go into the spa industry. So when she made the move, she told me, "Hey Tonya, I've got this spa down here and I don't have a clue what I'm doing. Can you come down here and help me out?"

I went down, I went in, and I saw that she really didn't have any idea of how to run a spa. I mean she has business sense, but she didn't understand the ins and outs of how a spa works. I decided to help, and I was able to apply that experience to my degree plan.

I totally went to work. First I helped her put together a strong team of professionals for massage therapy. I hired them, I trained them, I taught them everything I know. I taught them the maybe twelve methodologies I knew for massage–Swedish, deep tissue, shiatsu, reflexology, you name it–I taught them skin care, massage therapy, body wraps, everything. I helped put together the menu of services, I helped her understand what kinds of treatment rooms she needed, how to order products so that she never ran out and so she never overstocked, how to make the spa a real experience, just like it had been when I worked for Steven Deer. Then once everything was ready, we went through a marketing campaign where we had story layouts in some of the biggest magazines in Dilworth.

We turned around and made it real boutiquish and very exclusive so when people came to visit, they felt like it was all for them. It wasn't a conveyor belt where you come in and you get your hair done and you get your makeup and you're out of there as soon as you arrive. It was an experience. An *Elite Experience*.

It was also a hands-on experience for me, too. It allowed

me to take all the things I had learned from my time in the beauty industry and train people with all of those things I knew. I helped them reinvent that whole spa, so much so that it became one of the top spas in Dilworth.

I was flying back and forth for that whole semester, almost every two weeks. I was always by myself, too, with only my cane to help me get around. It was a little daunting at first, but I got used to it. And the cool part about flying while being blind was that no matter what class I ordered, the airlines would always put me in first class because of my visual impairment. It was a nice perk. It made me feel a little safer going back and forth.

Another trip I took was with the Center for Vision Loss. We went to South Dakota to camp and visit Mt. Rushmore. It was my first camping experience, and let me tell you, it was *awesome*.

The campground was close to Mt. Rushmore and I was really scared at first. I was like, "Oh my God, we're gonna tough it out with no showers, no water, no nothing!? Oh my God, I don't know what this is going to be like!" I didn't have to worry too much though because when we got to the campground, we actually did have a bathroom to shower in. It was a mile away, but still. It was a *shower*!

We also had an opportunity to camp outside underneath the stars and make s'mores around the campfire. We ate berries and nuts and all sorts of natural food. There was one day where I stayed behind in the tent and the squirrels started to come around. They were looking at me like, "How you doing, Tonya? You gonna feed me?" It was just so beautiful. I didn't realize how much I loved nature until I had the opportunity to go camping and really experience it. I fell in love with the outdoors.

Now, it wasn't rainy, it wasn't cold, it wasn't any of that. It was sunny, with absolutely beautiful weather the whole time. That might've been why I enjoyed it so much.

There was a pond you could kayak in at the campground. We'd get in this little boat and we'd kayak and it was during one of those kayaking trips where I saw an eagle for the first time—and believe me, as a visually impaired person, I *saw* the eagle. I mean his wings were stretched so wide, as big as the windshield of a car. We were in the boat, kayaking around the pond, and there was a tree over off to the right. It's right at the edge of the pond, with some of its branches over the water, but way up at the top there's this nest. We couldn't see the babies, but you could hear them all right! The little baby eagles inside were going, "Squawk squawk squawk! Squawk squawk squawk!" And meanwhile, we're still going toward it!

Not a good idea.

My partner explained how there was a baby eagle ahead and that that was what we were hearing. All of a sudden, the momma bird swoops down like *WHOOSH*. She flew right over us and glided on over to her nest up in that tree. My partner was like, "Well, Tonya, you wanna get closer?"

"No way," I told him. "Call me wimp, call me punk, call me whatever, but you take me and put me back on land because I'm pretty sure she's gonna do whatever it takes to protect her baby if we get any nearer."

That trip was full of great experiences like that. I got a

chance to play my flute amongst the trees, climb Mount Rushmore all the way up and all the way down, and we even went into caves deep underground. I got to collect different crystals and beautiful rocks and rose quartz–all just coming straight out of the ground! It was *so* awesome, just like when I went to Sapelo Island and I collected seashells off the beach. I'd clean them off and keep them as keepsakes.

When I first lost my vision, I never thought I'd be able to do all of the traveling that I've done. It took me a while, but I learned that there *is* life after blindness. Just because you have a physical challenge doesn't mean your life is over. Everybody's got challenges. You may not be able to see it, but we all have our own particular challenges that we're dealing with. And a challenge doesn't mean you give up on life. It doesn't mean you should be bitter for the rest of your life. It doesn't mean you stop living. It means you push through and enjoy life. You either let your challenges roll over you and you give up, or you say, "I'm going to fight kicking and screaming, and while I'm at it, I'm going to have a good time." I try to enjoy life to the fullest because I'm here for a reason. I'm here for a purpose, and evidently, my time is not up. So until that day comes, I'm going to make the best of it.

I took that philosophy with me everywhere I travelled. I don't think I really put it into action, though, until I went out of the country to study in Costa Rica.

7 | Study Abroad Gone Wrong

I've always wanted to travel. Whenever someone learned that about me though, they'd have this look on their face like, "Really?" People tend to think that because you're visually impaired, you can't do things. But you can. I had my own style, I was doing well living independently, I went shopping and I liked cooking and I went to school and I was living a "normal" lifestyle. And so the next step for me was to travel. I didn't care what anybody else thought. I wanted to see what it was like to go learn Spanish in a Spanish-speaking country.

I also liked being the first. I was the first visually impaired person to study abroad at Metro State.

I was excited. I was just totally excited. I was getting myself prepared, you know, buying the clothes, the supplies, counting down the days, all of it. This trip was going to be like a vacation for me. And I'd get to learn at the same time! A double whammy! Mixing my education with travel was fun for me–I've loved learning since I was a little girl. When I was putting the study abroad into my degree plan, I was like, "Oh, this is gonna be fun!"

I was most excited to learn all about a new culture. I've always been curious about different cultures. I have a lot of friends from different parts of the world and I've always asked them, "How do you say 'hi'?" and, "How do you say 'bye'?" and "How do you say 'thank you'?" Those are universal phrases that everyone should know in as many languages as you possibly can. I think when you run across people from different parts of the world and different walks of life, if you acknowledge them and their culture in *their* language, they are willing to help you more so than if you didn't try at all. And even if you're doing a butchered-up job at speaking their language, most of the time, if you're really genuine, the fact that you're trying is enough. It makes people happy when you're concerned enough to try to bridge that gap.

A lot of work was put into me going to Costa Rica. I had to get my books bought before I went on the trip so they could be translated and put into an audio format and then finally airmailed to me in Costa Rica. They issued me a driver instead of having me take the bus like everyone else because they needed to make sure I got back and forth to school. One struggle they weren't exactly able to accommodate was all my technology. It was difficult for them to translate their work into electronic format for me because the school in Costa Rica wasn't as tech-savvy as we are the States. That was a hurdle I thought was going to be a bigger struggle once I got there, but it turned out okay. I learned how to speak Spanish in other ways.

When I first got to Costa Rica, everyone was trying to be polite with me. They were trying to see how I fit in at the school, being visually impaired and everything. No one like me had studied abroad before. It was new for all of us, even the driver who took me to and from school. They hadn't needed a driver before.

My host family really enjoyed having me there. Everyone kept trying to figure out what I could actually see and what I couldn't. They wanted to know how I got around safely and how I walked and how I used my cane and how I did just about everything. I guess everyone just had to learn *me*—everyone being both my host family and the school staff.

The teachers and students and whatnot would greet me every day when I came in with the driver. He would walk me from the car to the main office and then I'd go by myself from the main office to wherever my classes were. The school was real interesting because our classrooms were kinda like in a bungalow or cabin style on these small hills, so when you would walk from one to another–aw man, you got some exercise in! I think my body was the tightest it's ever been in my life because I did so much walking up and down those hills. Up a hill, down a hill, over a hill, back and forth between the hills. Every day it was *a lot* of walking.

And so to go from one class to another class it would be a struggle! We'd start off in the homeroom, which is in the main house up front at the top of one of those hills. Then we'd walk down the hill to whichever bungalow your class was in. And if we had to go to the bathroom, well, that was all the way back at the top of the hill. By the end of the day, you're just panting, completely out of breath.

Everybody was kinda standoffish at the beginning, everyone except my host family. I really loved them like they were my own family. My host mama was so sweet and so kind. One time she took me into town and out to lunch, just her and I. We had some pistachio ice cream and she took me to get our toes done, too. She had saved up her money for the treat. I thought it was just the sweetest.

Now my host papa, he was funny. One particular evening, I'm sitting on the porch and I come inside and Host Papa is in the TV room smoking a joint! I was like, "What the what!?" He's around sixty or seventy years old, just smoking away! He saw me and was like, "Yeah, this is earth, this is life!" I thought that was like the funniest thing I've ever seen. I've never seen somebody that old partake in that stuff and be cool with it.

It was nice to be treated like family. They were the friendliest people, and I know we're still friends even though I'm not down there anymore. That's a major lesson I took from Costa Rica: once you made a friend, you made a friend for life.

One of my friends for life was a guy named Eduardo. While everyone was being standoffish to me, I met him and his friend Calvin and they were super friendly with me. They met me and said, "Hey, how you doing? Wait a minute, you're visually impaired! And they've got you moving around all by yourself? Oh no, you're not gonna be alone. We've got you! We're gonna go ahead and you're gonna learn all about Costa Rica with us."

It was Day Two or Day Three when I met them and we stayed friends for the whole rest of the program. Eduardo was one of my classmates, but not from Minnesota. He actually went to Mississippi Valley State and his major was foreign language, so he was there just to live in the country and pick up the language. That was actually like his fourth trip so it was like a second home to him. Everybody knew Eduardo and Eduardo knew everybody. He and Calvin knew where all the cool places were, where all the good food was, where the best deals were, where you could go get your hair cut, where you could go shopping, where you could go party, where you could do anything you wanted–he knew everything. They were the perfect tour guides.

My host family and I lived in Carrillos Bajo, a town northwest of the country's capital, San José, and Eduardo lived in Carrillos Alto, right nearby. So most days, I would go to school and learn Spanish (since that was what I was there for), I would come home from school, and then my friend Eduardo would come get me so we could go explore. Usually we went into San José, the capital of Costa Rica, or go out to experience Costa Rica's luscious environment.

I really enjoyed when Eduardo would take me into San José. He would escort me everywhere because he thought someone should be with me instead of just dropping me off at school by myself. And when we went places together, that's how I learned how to speak Spanish. It was difficult to learn a new language without my technology, but Eduardo and Calvin would purposefully take me into town, into the culture, so I could catch onto the language more quickly just by immersing myself in the Costa Rican lifestyle—and so I could get a taste for the food! It was all really great. I truly enjoyed the authentic Latin food. *Gallo pinto. Pescado. Cerveza.* It was so tasty—and cheap! We pay a fortune for all that here, but there it's really inexpensive. And believe it or not, it was the fast food that we're familiar with in the States that was the expensive stuff. McDonald's is like going to maybe a Smith and Wollensky's Steakhouse in Costa Rica. It's a big deal.

Oh, the food was just so good! Every morning, my host mom would fix me all sorts of meals. *Gallo pinto* with a salad and some fruit, *pescado* with a sweet roll, coffee as good as any Starbucks back home! (Of course, Costa Rica is where they get their beans!) Then when she was finished cooking, she would sit and have breakfast with me too.

My host papa was a semi driver, so he would come back to the States every once in a while and drive, and then he would bring his money home and convert it. His job allowed the family to live comfortably. They had this really beautiful and really big villa, with two bathrooms, four bedrooms, ceramic tiles all along the floor, and lots of open windows. No panes, no glass, just screens you could close so there was always ventilation coming in.

Everything is just so different down there. Costa Rica is a very eco-friendly country. A very clean and very neat culture. Like, when you would go to the bathroom, you weren't supposed to put toilet paper in the toilet. You put it in the garbage can and they'd tie it up and toss it out every night and clean everything down and it's not stinky or anything. They have strict rules with water, making the water so fresh that you don't need bottled water or an extra filter. You can literally drink water out of the tap or a fountain and it's eco-friendly. It's not contaminated. Or like when you take showers, you only have so many minutes to get your shower done with hot water before it goes cold. It's to preserve the water. When I first heard of that, I thought it was so weird because I've never lived like that. I was like, "Oh wow, what do you mean I can't take a thirty-minute hot shower? What do you mean I can't put the toilet paper in the toilet? Are you serious?" It was a lot to get used to, but after a while, I started to like it.

Another difference was the Internet cafés. Costa Rica is so off the grid–though I don't know if it's changed since I was there almost nine years ago now–but people don't have Internet or a wireless connection at home like a lot of people do in the states. Instead, you go to these Internet cafés and that's where you go to do your work. They're like a real big money-maker.

Paper products are expensive there too. It's an odd commodity. One day I went into a store with my host family and while they were grocery shopping, I grabbed a couple notebooks without looking at the price. They were just little composition notebooks, so I didn't think nothing of it. I figured they were only like a dollar ninety-nine a piece. So we get to the cash register and I'm expecting my bill to come out to maybe ten, fifteen dollars. I'm really savvy when it comes to spending money. I usually know what I'm going to pay before the register is finished ringing. Well, my bill came out to sixty plus dollars. Yeah, for just a couple notebooks!

I got upset. I was like, "No no no no, you're cheating me!"

What I didn't recognize then was that Costa Ricans have very agreeable spirits. Nobody ever says no. They just smile and say yes. Even if they don't want to, they'll say yes. So when I challenged the cashier and asked him to recount my total, it was really offensive. I didn't understand what was going on. When my host parents started getting embarrassed, I think that was when I realized what I'd done. I got so embarrassed myself. They explained to me that each book was like seven dollars a piece. I could pay ninety-nine cents to a dollar ninety-nine back home.

"Put them all back," I said. I wasn't about to make that purchase.

A few days later, I came home from school and my host mama gave me a gift. It was a stack of paper just for me. With that stack of paper she gave me a book that talked all about Costa Rica and its rainforests and basically everything there is to know about the country. It was like a tourism book. It was so sweet! That's how sweet my host family was. It was like I was their daughter.

I loved going out to explore the country. One time, some of the other girls from campus and I went to Manuel Antonio Beach. We had a week to ourselves where we didn't have to worry about classes or school or anything! It was an awesome experience.

We took a looooong bus trip to the beach. It felt so long it was like we could have flown. Anyway, at this point in the study abroad program, I'm getting so tired of having to speak Spanish everywhere I go. I just wanted to get a chance where I could just cheat and speak a little English! Well, on this bus trip, I saw somebody who I thought might've been from the States. They looked exactly like me–our skin tones were the same. Back in Carrillos, no one looked like me. The person even looked like someone from back home that I knew. It kinda threw me off. So I went up to them and I said, "Man, how are you doing?"

They looked at me all confused and said, "*Qué?*"

I was so embarrassed! I was like, "Oh wow! I'm sorry. I mean, *lo siento.*"

So with all these different cultures, everyone speaks Spanish. Like, America is mixed with so many different shades and skin tones and cultures just like Costa Rica, but instead of speaking a whole bunch of different languages like in the States, everyone in Costa Rica speaks Spanish. It was really cool to see so many different cultures mixed up in one singular culture. Every person was truly a Costa Rican.

When we finally got off that bus, we found ourselves a nice place to stay off the beaten path. It was little hotel right by the beach. We'd go spend time out in the sun, right by the water, just relaxing. Oh, it was something special! The currents were so strong you couldn't swim in the water, but you could walk right on down and plant your feet at the water's edge and let the warm water just glide right up to your ankles. Oh, the water was as warm as a sauna! Like a spa. Each time I got my feet wet I was like, "Ah, this is the life!" You'd think the water would be ice cold being from the ocean and all, but it was actually really warm.

One of the funny things about that beach was they have these real pretty silver monkeys that climb around way up in the trees. Everyone always tells you, "Do not feed the animals!" And I didn't think nothing of it, but we watched and saw how the monkeys literally come all the way down and they snatch your purse, your camera, your technology, everything. It's like someone trained these monkeys or something. They snatch all your belongings and go right back up into the tree. And that's it. You never get your stuff back. They take it and go.

I was lucky. I had seen the monkeys come down, snatch some cameras and purses that belonged to some other people in the group and run right back up those trees. I was like, "Oh okay, I'm gonna hold everything *really* close now." The trees were so tall, too, that you couldn't even see the tops of them, so there's no way you can catch those monkeys and get your things back. It's not like if someone on the street grabs your purse where you can run after them. If the monkeys take your stuff, it's just gone.

So next time you're in Costa Rica, hold onto your belongings and don't get mesmerized by the cute little monkeys!

The shopping was phenomenal and awesome, too. Lots of things to buy and keep away from the monkeys. Everywhere you went the prices were extremely reasonable. I'm still kicking myself for not purchasing that hammock for five dollars. If I wanted to get one now, I'd probably have to pay at least two hundred dollars here in America for one.

We visited some cool places while at the beach, too. One of the most fun places was a nightclub. The music was a mixture of hip hop, reggae, and salsa–all together in the music.

I was like, "Wow, this is crazy! Is that Tupac? Oh my God, is that Bob Marley? Wait, is that–?" So it was really really interesting the way they mixed it in. It really sounded good. It really did. I'd never experienced a night like it before. And I haven't since then, either.

On our last night at the beach, we went to a place called *Sol Bajo*. "Sunset" in English, I think. It was an indoor and outdoor restaurant where you could either sit at a regular table on the inside or go outside and sit cross-legged on these big throw pillows at tables that were really low to the ground. The food there, like everywhere else in Costa Rica, was phenomenal. But the food–as amazing as it was–wasn't the best part of the restaurant. The best part was that while you're sitting there drinking your margaritas and eating your food and whatnot, you get to watch the sun go down over the water. While the sun is setting, you have fire throwers on the deck doing a whole routine: they're dancing, they're throwing fire around, music is playing. Visiting *Sol Bajo* was one of my biggest highlights during the trip.

I really loved the whole experience, so much so that I wanted to get dual citizenship. I was trying to figure out how to do it, but there weren't a whole lot of options. In order to be a dual citizen, you either have to get married to a native (of course, that's the number one way), open up a business in the country with at least one hundred thousand dollars, or go to school there, learn the constitution, take the test, and do it in Spanish, both written and verbally.

See, I did my research. I was really thinking about it!

It was just such an awesome experience. The beautiful

rainforests, the delicious food, all of the natural culture–I loved all of it. My only regret was that I never got a chance to taste the sugarcane.

+

My study abroad program got cut short. One morning I was going to class and my driver drove me in, like usual. Now, when you pull into the campus, you have to go up this hill. My driver parked the car on the hill, and me being trained as a child to never walk in front of a car and always walk behind it instead so the driver doesn't go forward and accidentally hit you, I started walking behind it to get inside. I was a little confused, because this particular morning no one came out to greet me to make sure I got inside like they usually do. So when my driver was getting ready to go, I was walking around the back. He didn't see me because I was lower than him–we're on a hill, remember–so he backed up and he hit me.

I go flying into the air. I don't know how many feet up it was, but it felt like a lot. I had the technology I was able to get at the school on a dolly beside me, and when I got hit I was holding onto it. Because of that dolly, I landed back down on my feet. If it wasn't there, I don't know what would have happened to me.

So I get hit by the car. I'm startled. I'm scared. I'm glad to be alive. All the above. The driver got out of his car and some of the school officials came out of the building when they heard what happened and everyone was like, "Are you okay? Are you okay?"

I'm like, "Yeah, yeah, I'm fine." Everyone goes their separate ways.

Twenty minutes later though and the adrenaline rush had left. Then I was like, "Oh, I'm in so much pain. I don't feel good. I need to go to the hospital."

When I talked to the director of the program, they were like, "Oh no. You can't go to the hospital."

I was shocked. I was like, "What?"

"You didn't take the ambulance so you can't go."

"Well, I got insurance in case of an emergency before I came down here. I need to go to the hospital."

But still, they said, "No no no, it's going to cost you five hundred American dollars if you want to go to the hospital."

I was getting real scared. "What happened to the insurance that I purchased before I came over here with this program?"

"Oh, that doesn't count. You cannot go to the hospital."

"But I'm hurt."

They just weren't going to let me go. It didn't make sense. It was dangerous, I was in a lot of pain, it felt like a big truck hit me, not just a small car. I think they were probably more concerned about the possibility of getting sued. I don't know. It just didn't make any sense to me.

I went home early and my host mom was absolutely furious. But she technically couldn't do anything either. My host family was hired by the school, so they could have lost their contract if they didn't do what the school told them to do–and the school told them not to take me to the hospital. My host mom was so upset though that she got me in a cab and took me into town to see a doctor anyway.

We went to a clinic since the school told me I couldn't go to a hospital, so they didn't really have any sophisticated equipment. The doctor was only able to give me pain medicine. He wanted to make sure nothing was broken, but they couldn't do X-rays so all the doctor could do was check for any protruding bones. Obviously he didn't find any. I would've known if I'd had any bones sticking out like that. He just checked my vitals and gave me something for pain so I could rest.

What I was really worried about were the blood clots. They couldn't do those tests there at that clinic, and the school wouldn't let me go to a hospital, so I realized I had to get back to the States. I had to make sure my clots weren't traveling as a result of that accident.

I was in so much pain that I couldn't go to school the next day. When I didn't show up, they had the audacity to come to the house and ask, "Why didn't you come to school today?"

It was unbelievable. I was like, "Um, news flash. I got hit by a car yesterday and you wouldn't let me go to the hospital."

Of course, they felt like I was being insubordinate. It just became a nightmare really quick then. The school told everyone I knew that they couldn't talk to me, including my friends who would take me into town every day. It was really really bad. I think they were scared that they were going to be sued and if people contacted me there would be even more problems, so they were doing everything they could to make sure they weren't gonna lose money, instead of being more concerned about my health and wellness. It was really sad.

They were keeping my friends from me and they weren't

letting me get the medical help I needed. What I needed was to go home to make sure I didn't get another blood clot from the accident. But the school wouldn't send me back home, even though I kept telling them, "I need to go back home to see my doctors because I had a previous blood clot. I got hit by that car and I gotta make sure no more clots have arrived from that."

They didn't want to give me a ticket to go back home. The counselor here in America knew how dangerous my situation was. She knew about my previous blood clots. She knew they could be life-threatening if I didn't get checked out. So she took her own personal money and purchased me a ticket so I could get back home safely and go see the doctor. I felt bad because she ultimately got fired for this extreme act of kindness.

The day I was ready to leave, the school came to my host family's house and told me that my taxi couldn't take me anywhere until I signed a release form that said the school had no involvement in the situation and that I would not sue them. I was flabbergasted!

"Oh, you've got to be kidding me," I said. "You want me to sign what? Okay, this is the part where I'm gonna call the embassy because you guys are really losing it."

The embassy kinda regulated the situation from that point. They were like, "What? What do you mean you can't go home? Well what's the name of the school?" They ended up getting me out of there and taking me to the airport. I never signed the paper, but I never sued them either. I just wanted to live and be okay! It was a shame that they were willing to put my life at risk all because of the chance they could be sued.

The whole ordeal put my host family in a real compromising position. They didn't know what to do. And by the time the school officials let me go and I got to the airport, I had missed my flight. They made me miss my flight! The counselor had used her own money to get me out of there and they made me miss it! Oh, I was so mad. My counselor ended up calling the school, calling the airport, and getting me on another flight. The airport was kind enough to put me up in a hotel overnight. It was just a huge mess.

When I finally got back to the states, I got my test and I was clear of blood clots. I was fine in that department, but I was still having problems with the school. It was like problems on top of problems on top of more problems! They weren't going to refund me my money, they turned all of my classes into incompletes–which then turned into F's–and to top it all off, that's when the counselor discovered I'd written my Master's into my undergrad behind her back.

My counselor over the degree plan was an awesome lady. Unfortunately, she was on another sabbatical writing a book once I had returned from Costa Rica. So instead of going to her to sort out my degree plan, I met with the same lady who had told me I couldn't write my Master's into my undergrad. I only had a few more classes I needed before it was time for me to graduate–one more semester–but when the lady looked at my degree plan and she saw that I had taken classes for my Master's, she was absolutely ticked off.

She said, "I thought I told you that you could *not* take any of these classes!"

"Well," I tried to explain, "the course catalog said that I could take these classes with professor's permission and I got permission from every professor I ever dealt with."

She just wasn't listening. "Oh, we have a problem. We have a *huge* problem."

She contacted my professors, my counselor, the president, she probably contacted everyone at that school. It was very escalated. She told them I was a troublemaker, I was insubordinate, I was out of line. She tried to get me suspended from school. I had to go to all these people outside of Metro State to get help so I could stay. I went to Senator Betty McCullom and the National Federation for the Blind. My mother was a part of the NAACP at the time, so NAACP helped me as well. All three of them worked diligently to make sure that my rights as a visually impaired student weren't taken advantage of, and seeing that I kept such a high GPA–before they'd turned my grades to F's and dropped my 3.8 to like a 2.6–and was injured by circumstances beyond my control, it wasn't fair to kick me out of school. I still had the right to graduate and walk across that stage. And I got to do just that.

Even with all of the trouble that came out of it, I don't regret my trip to Costa Rica. My host family was full of loving people, I loved the culture, the people were so very friendly, the food was phenomenal, the language was fun to learn, everything was eco-friendly, very clean, very neat, very very beautiful, and in general, all the good during the trip outweighed the bad at the end by a lot.

But then things started to get worse, just like after my last great travelling experience at Sapelo Island.

8 | Paralyzed

When I got back from Costa Rica, I went to see a doctor as soon as I hit the landing strip to make sure I didn't have any clots. I was okay in the clot department, but I started having problems with my hip.

I didn't notice them right away. It was a few weeks after I got home, but I'm pretty sure the issues I had were related to the accident in Costa Rica. The pain was on my left side, even though I'd been hit on my right. My hip would pop in and out a lot, and I guess the accident must have shifted my body and affected the other side or something. I don't know for sure. I just know that whenever it would hurt, I would go to get it adjusted at a chiropractor.

I went to an office called Caron Chiropractic and told them I didn't know what was going on. I didn't know if it was a pinched nerve or something else, so they gave me an adjustment. Instantly I felt better. I was like, "Oh, yes!"

In hindsight, I wish I would've known better because I could've just stretched and that alone would've popped my hip right back into place instead of me having to continuously get it adjusted. Well, on one particular day, I went to the chiropractor to get my hip adjusted, no problems at all. I'd gone to him several times and there were never any issues. For some reason, when he adjusted me on this particular day, something went wrong. The procedure started out normal: he adjusted my head, he adjusted my spine, he was working his way down, but before he could get to my hip, my L2 or L3 (one of the spinal vertebrae in my lower back) was a little stiff. So he forced it and there was a pop.

I looked at him. He looked at me. We'd both heard it. And then he just says, "Okay, well you're done!"

The chiropractor didn't even get a chance to adjust my hip. I think he realized something was wrong so he stopped right away. I got up and was a little worried. I was just like, "Okay..."

He told me, "Well, do some stretches and you'll be fine. I'll see you next week. You've got an hour before you get your massage."

Normally, I didn't get massages after an adjustment. I had a lot of stress on my plate at the time though and so I thought I'd go ahead and get one. Usually I would go to my friend Celeste for a massage. I'm very finicky about who I let do a massage for me since I did massage myself, but at the time, the chiropractor was giving out free massages. A super deal, right? Well, everything free is not always good.

With the time I had, I decided to go across the street to a

bar and grill. I wanted some of my favorite criss-cross fries with a mild barbecue sauce. On my way over there, though, I felt like my equilibrium was off. I sat down and it got a little better, so I ate my fries and just relaxed, and then when I was on my way back to the chiropractor's, I was literally walking side to side, trying to stay balanced. I was just thinking, *Oh wow, this is not good.*

Before I went to do the massage, I returned to the chiropractor and told him, "You know, something's just not right. I think something's wrong with my hip."

He said, "Well, okay, I'll tell the massage therapist what you need and you should be all right."

I thanked him and went in for my massage. I wasn't sure if he was right but I went ahead with it anyway. I don't really like to tell people about my credentials because it makes people nervous sometimes. If I tell the masseuse, "You know I'm a massage therapist and I've done this for seventeen years and I have all this experience and I think it should be done this way and yada yada yada," it makes them tense and you can feel that in the massage. You won't experience what you really want to experience: a relaxing massage.

Well, I thought it was going to be relaxing, but it was very aggressive, even without me speaking up. It was a deep tissue massage, but she was going *way* too deep. She wasn't supposed to be going that deep. What a lot of people don't know is that if you're getting a deep tissue massage–or any massage, for that matter–it doesn't necessarily have to hurt. If it hurts, just tell your massage therapist, "It hurts." Then they can lighten up.

I told the masseuse a couple times and she lightened up a

little, enough so that I could fall asleep. Whenever I get myself on that table, I have a really bad habit of falling asleep. No matter what, I just zonk out! Maybe because I don't sleep enough at night or something, I really don't know. But I fell asleep, she continued the massage, and when we were finished, I was sore *all over*.

I told her I was sore but she just kinda shrugged it off. She was like, "Oh yeah, drink a gallon of water and it'll help. You're going to be sore for a couple of days."

I knew what kind of soreness I should've been feeling, and this was a lot worse. I was like, "Oh, I'm gonna be back."

I was so sore! When I got home, I could feel pressure going from my heart all the way down my arm, right up into my hand. I was like, "Am I having a stroke? Am I having a heart attack?"

It was awful. I was scared, too, because I'm always cautious about my heart and veins and whatnot because of the blood clots I had in my lungs.

I tried a home remedy when I couldn't take it any longer. I often make this yummy concoction with cayenne pepper, lemon, and honey. It's supposed get the blood flowing and then I'd be okay. You just mix together like a tablespoon of cayenne pepper, a little bit of honey, and a squeeze of lemon juice in hot water, drink that, and it stops a heart attack or a stroke. It opens up your arteries and it flushes your blood all through your body. It's a lifesaver. It's an old remedy–or I should say a holistic or natural remedy–but it's a lifesaver nonetheless.

But this time, it wasn't doing anything. So I called the

emergency room and asked, "Hey, I'm just checking, but my chest hurts a little bit, the pain goes all the way down my left arm, and I don't feel it on my right. Do I need to come in?"

They were like, "Oh, you need to come into the emergency room right now."

"I'm on my way."

I went straight to the emergency room, and right around this time there was something going on in Minnesota where they had shut down all insurance policies so the doctors didn't want to do any major tests or anything. The whole budget for federal workers and everything was frozen. How convenient for me, right? So everything was frozen when I went to the emergency room and when someone came to examine me, they were just like, "Oh, take two aspirin and call us in the morning."

I was really upset. I was like, "What? Okay, I see what this is. You don't want to run a test to see if my clot has traveled to my heart or anything? Oh, I get it." I was *really* upset. "I won't be back."

So I get home, I take my two aspirin, and the pain is back again the next day. I couldn't bear it, so I called the owner of the chiropractor's office. I told him, "I just want to let you know that your intern adjusted me and then I got a massage that was so rough I had to go to the emergency room. I can't breathe, I'm in so much pain, and this and that and the other thing."

He said, "Why don't you come in and I'll see what I can do for you."

So I went back to the chiropractor's and the owner did

something where he used a laser and then put Kinesio Tape on me. When he put on the Kinesio Tape, I didn't have any problems with my breathing. It felt amazing! The Kinesio Tape was keeping my pain intact so I could function, but whenever the Kinesio Tape would come off–like when I would take a shower–well, guess what? The pain came right back all over again.

I needed a permanent fix, but instead of going back to the emergency room, I decided to go to a clinic. I thought that I wouldn't be having a heart attack for this long, so they might be able to help me.

At first the doctors there didn't believe me. I kept insisting that I could possibly have a blood clot and it could have traveled to my lung again. They still didn't want to run the test. In order to discover if you've got a blood clot, you've got to do a CAT scan. They were just like, "Well, how do you *know* you have a blood clot?"

I was like, "I've had one before and it feels similar to that. I was hospitalized for it previously so I need to get it checked out."

They were like, "Well, do you think that maybe this is something you think is occurring that isn't actually occurring?"

"Uh, no. That's why I'm here: to make sure I don't drop dead."

"Well, maybe we should give you some medication to calm you down. It's antipsychotic, and maybe we can sit you down with a counselor if that would help."

I think they were thinking I was a hypochondriac because I had been to the clinic several times but they couldn't find anything wrong with me since they didn't want to do the tests. They thought my pain was all in my head. They literally had to roll me into the building in a wheelchair from the cab and they still thought I was just making it up.

And then when they brought up the antipsychotics I knew I wasn't gonna be getting anywhere. I was sharp. I knew what was happening. I was like, "Oh, I see where this is going. There's nothing wrong with me mentally. I don't know why you're trying to give me antipsychotic medication for this. I'm telling you: there's something going on with my chest and my arms and my hands."

But they couldn't figure out what it was. And because they couldn't figure out what it was, they wanted to give me some antipsychotic medication. I told them no to the antipsychotics and they said the most they could do was give me some valiums for the pain. I took those and I left. I didn't want to deal with them anymore if they weren't gonna help me.

That's the thing about the medical industry. If you want to say no to something–a procedure, a test, an examination, whatever–you have that right to say no. I said no then, and I left.

I called my friend Celeste. I'd done massage therapy for seventeen years, Celeste had been doing it for twenty-one at that time. She was really good at what she did. She's the one I would normally go to if I needed a massage, prior to all this happening. And she knew me, my demeanor, my mindset, everything. She knew I didn't need antipsychotics. So I called her and I said, "Uh, Celeste?"

"Yeah Tonya?"

"I need to come see you."

"Oh, yeah sure, c'mon!"

"Uh, well, I'm in real bad shape."

"I'm sure you can't be that bad! We'll figure it out."

"Okay, I'm just letting you know."

So I got a cab and I went straight to her from the clinic. And I was like barely standing up. The cab driver was scared that I was gonna fall and he was worried about liability issues. I got there safe and sound, but when I got out of the cab, I struggled.

Celeste's studio, Celestial Touch, is connected to a really popular café in Saint Paul called "Golden Thyme". They'd host poetry readings, live music, all sorts of stuff. It was a real cultural hotspot there in Minneapolis, and so in order to get to her studio, you have to go in through the café with all these people eating and hanging out and stuff. Well, I got out of the cab and I walked into the café and everyone just looked at me like, "You need some help? Are you okay?" Everyone was afraid I was gonna fall. That's how bad I was walking. Looking back, I can't even believe they would let me leave the clinic like that.

Finally I got to Celeste's studio and she was very calm about the whole situation. She said, "Oh. Well, okay. Tonya. Tell me what's happening." She made me feel really comfortable. I wasn't scared going to her.

I said, "Well, what happened was I got an adjustment and I heard my back pop. And then I got this massage and, oh my God, it was the worst massage ever. She was really rough, really *really* rough."

Celeste was an expert. She knew what it was right away. She told me, "Oh, okay so that's what it is. Nine times out of ten, it's your thoracic muscle that's been irritated in cases like this, so it's the one causing spasms. She overworked your thoracic muscle. It's one of the largest muscles in the body. It wraps around your ribs near your heart and comes down toward your waist, so if you're having contractual spasms in that muscle, it feels like you're having a heart attack. It's cutting off your breathing."

I knew going to Celeste was a good idea!

Then she asked, "Okay, what did they give you?"

"They gave me some valiums."

"Yeah, you need to take 'em. You also need to go home, put on some relaxing music, meditate, and rest. Tonya, I know you're a workaholic. You can't be your normal self right now. I need you to rest and heal."

I was real appreciative of Celeste's help. I told her I would take it easy and then I headed out.

Before I made it home, I stopped by the chiropractor's office again. I needed more Kinesio Tape. I went back to the owner and said, "Look. I need to *buy* some of your Kinesio Tape. I figured out what was wrong and I need it so I don't have to keep coming back here to put it on while I'm recovering."

He didn't really want to sell me any. "Well, you need to be trained and—"

"No no no no," I said. I wasn't gonna take no for an answer. "I *need* some of that Kinesio Tape before I go home." Celeste had told me to go home and rest, and I couldn't rest if those spasms kept continuing. I needed some more Kinesio Tape to mute the pain.

Now, when I walked into the chiropractor's office, all the patients in the lobby looked at me like I was some monster because I couldn't walk. The therapists were like, "We've got clients in here. We can't have you coming into the office like this, making us look really bad and everything!" They didn't want me scaring away patients, so ultimately the owner decided to sell me some Kinesio Tape. I was really happy about that.

Before I left, I told the owner, "Well, I'll call you guys and let you know what happens." That was the last time I ever saw them, though. I never gave them that call.

When I got home, I fell. I didn't have the Kinesio Tape on yet, and I was walking down the hallway with both arms holding onto the wall so I could keep my balance. Well, I lost that balance and I couldn't get up. My mom tried to help me up and it took all of her power to get me up on the chair. Before when we went to the clinic, she wasn't so sure about my pain either. She thought I might've needed those antipsychotics. So when I fell, I asked her, "Now do you believe something's wrong?"

She was like, "Yeah, something's wrong."

We went to the emergency room, this time I going to a different hospital: United. They went through the usual questioning: "Are you vulnerable? Is anybody abusing you? What medications do you take? Any reason why this might be happening that you can recall?"

I told them, "Nobody's abusing me, I'm not on any medication, but you know what, I did get the strongest massage I've ever had the other day."

The doctors were like, "Okay then, we gotta run some tests and make sure that they didn't break anything in your spine from too much pressure."

So they ran a series of tests on me. They gave me all these crazy tests, telling me that the blood clots in my lungs were travelling to my heart. We were focused on the blood clots and not my ability to walk. In the mean time, my walking was getting worse and worse and worse.

And so for one of the tests, the doctors took me to this room where there was this big metal round machine in the ceiling, and attached to this machine was like this long cylinder with a point on the end, almost like a giant needle. That was supposed to go in my spine. It comes down and pricks you, real simple. It didn't look simple, though. It looked like something out of a torture chamber.

They were pulling me into the room and I was like, "What is that? What's that gonna do to me?"

They told me, "We're about to take this test called a lumbar puncture where we retrieve some cerebrospinal fluid from your spine. It's a regular test, completely standard, nothing to worry about."

I wasn't so sure about that. I said, "Um, no. I don't think I want to do this."

"Well, you already signed for it, so we have to do this test, Miss Rabb."

"Oh, I don't think I want to take this test anymore though."

"But your doctor ordered it."

"No, I don't think I need this."

"But don't you want to know why you're not walking? This test can help figure that out."

"I'm walking with assistance, but I don't think I want to do this one."

They weren't going to take no for an answer. "Oh, Miss Rabb, you have to take this test. It's required."

"Nope. Nope. Nope nope nope. I do not want to do this."

We went back and forth about it for a good ten/fifteen minutes. When they got tired of me saying no, they just went against my wishes and did the procedure anyway. They lowered the side of the gurney, rolled me over, held my arms and legs down, and punctured my spine.

It wasn't pleasant. It didn't feel good. It was painful. I just couldn't stop thinking about how they were holding me down. It couldn't possibly be legal. I had no one there to protect me, no one there to stop it, and they were doing it against my will. It was a really scary experience.

Once they got the fluid, they rolled me back over and said, "Don't move for six hours." They said they needed to get the cerebrospinal fluid from my spine but really it just seemed like a torture experiment to me.

Later, I came to find out that this test was one where you're supposed to be balled up, knees to your chest. They laid me flat on my stomach. I don't know if it was because they were forcing me or what, but that wasn't how the test was supposed to go. After it was over, they rolled me back onto the gurney and told me, "Don't move for six hours or you'll be paralyzed."

Six hours later I couldn't feel anything from my waist down.

+

I don't know what it was exactly that made me lose the use of my legs. It might've been that test, it might've been the pop at the chiropractor's, it might've been the deep massage I had, I don't know. It could have been a combination of all three that did it to me. All I know is that after those six hours, I couldn't feel anything from the waist down. Not my legs, not my feet, not even my little toes.

On top of that, I started having chest pain. I couldn't breathe. I was crying because my chest was hurting so bad. I was like, "I can't breathe, I can't breathe." My chest felt really heavy and the next thing I knew, I passed out. I think I flatlined.

When I woke up, they were pulling me out of an elevator. We had moved floors. There were a lot of people around my stretcher. It was really fuzzy, and I passed back out.

When I woke up again, I was on the cardiac floor with all these machines around me and a heparin drip in my arm. There was a doctor there with me and he said, "I did this to you." That was all I remember, because I passed out a third time.

The next time I woke up I stayed awake. I was in a different room with the heparin drip still in my arm. The blood clots had traveled to my heart. The heparin drip was forcing them out, so I was coughing up huge pieces of clots. It was scary.

While I was going through all the earlier procedures, I had a real sharp neurologist. She knew her stuff. She would just march in and she'd tell you what she needed to tell you and look directly at you and just walk back out because she just knew her stuff like that. Very confident, very to-the-point.

Well, this time around, that sharp neurologist came in and her whole disposition was different. It was like night and day. Her shoulders were curled, her head was down, she looked like she was unsure of herself. She sat down next to my bed and, with her head looking to the floor, said, "Um. You have something called Devic's."

I'm like, "What the hell is Devic's?"

"It's something very new."

"Something very new?"

"Yeah, something similar to multiple sclerosis, but it's not."

"How did you come up with that?"

"You've got Neuromyelitis optica, so–"

They were trying to tie this paralysis into my vision loss diagnosis from Georgia. But, remember, when I lost my vision, the optometrist didn't really know what was wrong with me, and so he gave me that diagnosis without fully knowing. He thought it could have been hysteria blindness, but I'm assuming he didn't diagnose me with that because it wouldn't have qualified for disability.

So because of that misdiagnosis, the sharp neurologist told me, "Well, according to your records in Georgia, you have Neuromyelitis optica. Devic's is related, and because you're not walking, that means you have it."

I didn't want to believe it. I was like, "Nuh uh. I walked in! I was barely walking, but I *walked* in. What do you mean I have Devic's? You know who did this to me? The chiropractor did this to me."

I was furious. They ended up bringing in a rehab doctor. I said, "So you're gonna rehab me?"

She was like, "Oh no no no no. I'm not touching you. You don't qualify for our program."

What was even the point of bringing in the rehab doctor if she wasn't gonna rehab me? "What do you mean I don't qualify for your program? The chiropractor did this to me and—"

"Nuh uh, the chiropractor didn't do this to you."

"What do you mean?"

"The chiropractor did not do this to you."

I think she was basically saying, "*We* did this, but I'm not going to say we did this." All she said to me was, "We're not rehabbing you."

She didn't want to touch me with a ten-foot pole because she knew what really was going on. I was upset with her when in reality she was trying to do me a favor. She was trying to tell me to put two and two together—that the chiropractor didn't do this to me, but that the hospital had. That's why she didn't want to rehab me. She didn't want to get caught up in the malpractice. But I wasn't seeing that. I was going through all these different emotions so I wasn't catching on to what she was telling me.

After the rehab doctor left, the neurologist came back in

and she was looking at the ground and she said, "We need to do this procedure for you."

"What procedure is that?"

"Well, we take all your blood out and we clean it and put it back in."

"That sounds like dialysis."

"Well yeah, it's kinda like dialysis but it's not."

I said, "What do you mean it's not? Can you explain that to me?" I wanted to be one hundred percent sure of all the tests I was gonna do from then on. I didn't want to be forced into nothing I didn't want to do.

"Well, I think I have a dialysis tech…"

"A dialysis tech!?"

"Yeah, I don't really understand the procedure."

I just looked at her, totally shocked and totally confused. I was like, "You don't understand the procedure, and yet you're telling me you need to do it? How many patients have you had like me?"

"You're the first."

Devic's was so new and so rare that I was United's first patient with it, and they had no idea what to do.

"Well, since you don't understand the procedure and I'm your first patient, I think I'll pass on that. Why don't you just send me somewhere I can get rehab? We'll do just fine."

She seemed real uncomfortable. She was still just looking at the floor, and she told me in a real quiet voice, "Okay, Ms. Rabb."

I've dealt with a lot of doctors, and what I've learned is that when they give you a diagnosis that isn't true, they automatically look at the ground. They don't look at you. They deliver the news facing down. But when they're telling you the truth, they're looking you dead in the face. They know it's the right diagnosis. I don't know if they're trained that way or if it's just an instinctual kind of thing, but it's something that happens.

This was the start of my life as a professional patient. What I mean by that term is someone who knows hospital politics and how to make sure they're getting the right treatment. You know how to watch your medications, you know the mannerisms of hospital staff and how you should talk to people, you know to have all your requests ready–maybe like eight or nine of them all at one time–so when a nurse finally answers your light, you can run down your list so you don't have to keep calling for each and every little thing. You know how to keep up with your vitals, how to note the medications you're taking, how to take everything a doctor tells you with a grain of salt because you can't trust every doctor who treats you and that you should always get a second opinion.

(I'm not saying all doctors are bad, but don't be so quick to sign off on every test they want to give you. They might say, "You need this, you need that," and you never question it. You should.)

You know that you've got two bookends of insurance: if you have really good insurance they can sometimes find things to be wrong with you so they can do all these expensive procedures or prescribe you with certain medications where they get a commission so they can make money off of your illness, or you don't have really good insurance and no one wants to treat you–and when you do get treated, you may not be able to pay for it. It's a scary world.

You know that you've got to have someone there with you whenever you have to go to the hospital. You should have a loved one right beside you who's always taking notes and always writing down the medications you're taking and the dosages and the terminology and the tests and the severe side effects and *everything*. You should be aware if a certain medication is going to shut down your liver eventually or do this or do that. You should know if you might develop symptoms from your medications so that they've got to give you more medication to clear up the symptoms that were created by the original medication in the first place. Next thing you know you're on twenty different medications and organs start failing.

Being in a hospital is not a hotel stay. Once you're in, don't just totally sign your life away. Pay attention, because you may never come out the same again. There are some doctors who are extremely good and know what they're doing, but there are some who aren't. Don't be so quick to say, "Okay." You say "okay" to one procedure and suddenly you're on a downward spiral and you're getting sicker and sicker and sicker and you don't know why.

That's exactly what happened to me.

9 | Norman

This massage accident wasn't the first time I'd found myself in the hospital. The only difference was that my first time, I was on the other side.

At one point in my life, early on in my marriage, my husband was ready for more kids. I had just received my cosmetology license, I was just starting my career, and my husband was like, "Okay, I'm ready to have more children!"

I just laughed. I was *not* ready! When I had carried my daughter, I was so huge that everyone thought I was having twins. I would waddle everywhere and everyone would be scared to take me places because they thought I was gonna pop at any time. And when I finally did have my daughter, I was in labor for twenty-four hours. It was a really rough, really difficult pregnancy for me. I was so young! I didn't want to go through that again, not right then anyway.

So I had to try to find a reason not to have another child. I told my husband, "Look. You went to school and you got your degree. I made sure you got your education first, so let me get my career off its feet and then we'll have another baby. How's that sound?"

He was okay with it. He said, "Okay. Well what do you wanna do?"

I was still so new to the cosmetology world that I didn't really know what I wanted to do in it, but I knew what I didn't want: another baby! So in my mind I was just thinking, *What career requires the most amount of time in school so that I can buy as much time as possible before I have another baby?*

So, naturally, I said, "I want to go to school to be a doctor!" I was just thinking all about those eight years in school and the three to five year residency afterward. Plus, being a doctor sounded pretty cool, so I decided to go with that.

I'm sure he was a little surprised, but he was supportive too. He told me, "Okay, well, Honey, if that's what you wanna do, that's what we'll do."

I landed a Certified Nursing Assistant (CNA) position at Rush Presbyterian-St Luke's in Chicago. I had received my certification beforehand while I was working at Gregory System–I was doing electrolysis, so you needed a certification for that–so they hired me right away. I was gonna climb my way up the hospital ladder, and I was able to get my foot in the door with that CNA license.

I worked with the surgical unit. I wanted to be a nursing anesthetist before I became a doctor, and that unit was where I could go to get my training. Rush also had an awesome program where if I worked full time, they would pay for my education to earn that degree. They were the only one in the state of Illinois that had a nursing anesthetist program like that.

It should have been right up my alley, right? Well, I had one fatal flaw: I cared too much.

My biggest weakness is compassion and caring. I have a really big heart and sometimes I try to hide it. When I found out that working in a hospital wasn't like *Quincy*–that television series about doctors who would take care of their patients with so much love and compassion and where everyone left with a good story–I had to get out of it.

One thing they always teach you in the medical industry is not to get attached to your patients because someone might pass away or something like that. But I couldn't be so cold to the patients. I mean, I would take care of each patient so good that the other nurses would come up to me and say, "Um, Tonya, you just splash some water on the patients and keep going. You don't need to go the extra mile. You're doing way too much."

I was totally appalled. I was young, I was passionate, I was too caring. I said, "Well, I have a grandmother and if anything happened to her, I would want someone to take care of her the way I'm taking care of these people. What goes around comes around and I think you're just out of pocket to tell me not to care for these people with the ultimate care!"

What I didn't realize was that I was setting standards for everybody else. If I was working above and beyond, if I was being way too caring than I should have been, then everyone else would have had to match me. And no one really liked that.

I was taking care of people like I was on *Quincy*, and the other nurses were like, "No, sweetheart, this is the real world. We're here to make money. We're not doing one-on-one health."

So I kinda got disengaged and disgruntled. They literally had to put somebody on top of me to make sure I wasn't taking care of the patients any more than what was required. They'd keep an eye on me and if I ever did more than I was supposed to, they'd tell me I was doing too much. I was making the other nurses look bad.

Medical work just wasn't what I thought it was.

By the time I wound up in the hospital again, I think I probably forgot a little about how hard nursing was.

When I left United, I went to this place called the Courage Center. The Courage Center is a nonprofit organization that helps people with disabilities win their independence back. I had been there before during my time at the University of Saint Paul because one of my teachers—who was just really awesome, I was really crazy about her—she also worked at the Courage Center in development, working with donors and gifts. At the time I was like, "I'm gonna come back here one day and work for you guys! I just graduated and got a Master's degree in non-profit organizational management and this is where I want to come work!"

The Courage Center had also given me a scholarship when I was going to school. I had written an essay about my blindness and how I was working to overcome the physical challenge to one day open my own wellness resort. They read my essay and gave me a pretty sizable scholarship for school. Then they brought me into the center, gave me a tour, I got to sit with a panel and ask them some questions, and it was just a really awesome experience.

So I had all these ties to the Courage Center, and instead of coming back to work for them like I'd wanted, I was back as a patient.

+

I was glad to go back. I thought the Courage Center was a good facility, they had helped me before, and one of the professors I really admired worked there—I thought it was the highest standard of rehab I could get. My only problem was that I didn't know about the politics of being a patient. I'd been on the other side before, but I wasn't thinking in terms of being a nurse. I was thinking in terms of being a patient, and I learned pretty quickly that there are just some things you have to let slide. You have to choose your battles carefully.

One thing I learned pretty quickly was that I had to be willing to wait. If you turn on your light or ring your bell and it takes the nurse forever to get to you, nine times out of ten they're taking care of other patients. It's not just you they have to worry about. They're doing their best to get to you. An emergency could have happened in another room. You don't know what else they have to deal with.

But that's difficult to learn at first. You're used to doing things for yourself and doing them right away. Instant gratification, you know? But it doesn't necessarily work that way when you have to depend on someone else to take care of you…and maybe six or seven people at the same time.

I should have learned sooner. I got assigned this nighttime nurse, but he was the extreme version of a bad nurse. He was terrible. He had this real blank expression, a stale monotone voice, and a very sinister attitude. He really creeped me out. He reminded me of Norman Bates.

The first night I was there, I told him, "I gotta go to the bathroom." Any other nurse would have helped me to the bathroom, let me go, and then helped me back to my bed.

But not Norman Bates. He just told me, "Oh, just pee on yourself and call me when you get done." And then he walked right on out.

I was like, "Okay, this is not cool." I rang the bell again and when he returned, I said, "Well, I have to *really* go to the bathroom." I didn't just have to pee, if you know what I mean.

"Oh, well, okay," he starts. I'm thinking now he's going to help me, but then he says, "Just have your bowel movement or whatever, ring the bell, and I'll come clean you up."

I'm going from a person who, normally, can get up and go to the bathroom if I gotta use the bathroom. If I gotta use the bathroom, I use it. There's not trouble. I'm not incognizant, I'm fully aware of when I gotta go, and so I shouldn't have to just go on myself. It was embarrassing. And so he told me this and I was like, "Oh no, who do you think you are? I'm gonna hold it. I'm not going on myself. I'm gonna hold this until you come back to get me."

But he never came back to get me. He was waiting for me to pee on myself. It was degrading. Completely humiliating.

So I wound up holding it all night. Prior to going to the Courage Center, I was also having issues with my digestive system. They'd worked really hard to get my digestive system going, but for me to say, "I'm not gonna go on myself so I'm gonna hold it all night," well, guess what? I just created the problem all over again.

When the daytime came, instead of just requesting another nurse–I didn't know I could do that–I reported him for negligent behavior. I didn't know the politics. I didn't know that they were going to just keep him on staff and that eventually I was gonna get him again. I should have stressed that I was uncomfortable with a man taking care of me, that I preferred to have a woman. That's your right as a patient. If you're a woman and you're not comfortable with a man taking care of you, you can request a female nurse. Plus, looking back on it, he kept trying to put me in situations where he would either have to wipe me, clean me, or catheterize me. Him putting me in these vulnerable situations as a man, when I was a woman. The whole situation seems a little messed up in hindsight.

So when the daytime nurse came in, I asked for the director of nursing and told her, "Well, I don't want him taking care of me no more. How would you like it if I told you that you can't use the bathroom and you either have to hold it until the next day or just go on yourself? Do you think that's fair?"

She was very professional with me. She was like, "Oh yes, yes, I see your dilemma."

I told her I didn't want him anymore. I wasn't thinking about what kind of skeleton crew they were working with, how understaffed they might be on the night shift. So, sure enough, two weeks later, I get Norman Bates again. This time, though,

I was ready. See, there was this machine I could stand on and the nurses could wheel me to the bathroom, wheel me to the shower, wheel me back to the bed, wheel me anywhere in my room. All it took was a simple push, and I could be anywhere they needed to roll me. So whenever I figured out that the nurse would be my nurse for the night, I developed a really bad habit. I'd ask whoever was my daytime nurse, "Can you just roll me into the bathroom and bring my tray? I know that when I'm done eating I'm gonna have to use the bathroom and I don't want to go on myself."

Yeah, it was pretty ridiculous. But that was my logic! I didn't want to go on myself.

So each time I got that nurse, he would do the same thing again and again where he didn't answer my calls the whole night. And so each morning, I reported him again to the nurse. She would say, "Oh, Miss Rabb, I'll make sure you don't have him anymore." But then two weeks later and there he is again!

Eventually, the nurses started straight catheterizing me. They did a bladder scan and said my bladder wasn't emptying fast enough, so that's why they had to straight catheterize me. Plus, they didn't want to get me up and take me to the bathroom each time I had to go. They felt it would have saved more time just to catheterize me. I wasn't too against this because then I wouldn't have to worry about going on myself anymore. So I went along with it. Instead of getting me in and out of the bed, the nurses would just catheterize me. That became the new routine.

Well, one particular morning, I had to go to court. When I was admitted into the hospital and I told them I had stairs, they wouldn't let me go home anymore. Whenever you are unable to walk and you have stairs in your home, oh, you can forget it. You're not going home. They won't let you go home until you can walk up stairs. It's not safe otherwise. How can you get up and down the stairs if you can't walk? You either need to be in a rehab facility or you need to be in a hospital, but you can't go home with stairs if you're not qualified to walk up them. So the last time I saw my home was before I went to the hospital. That's it. And I lost everything because of it.

I had to go to court because I was really upset with my landlord. When he found out I couldn't go home, he was going to evict me even though I was never late with the payments. I would always pay the rent on time and so I was absolutely appalled that he would even think to evict me. I was working on my health and I was going to get back there one way or another. I took it personally.

I didn't necessarily have to go to the court because I was in the hospital, but I felt like I needed to be there. This was my home! I wasn't just gonna let him evict me like that. So I went to the court date with an IV in my arm and everything. I didn't want to miss this date because I really wanted to look him in the face and be like, "Are you serious? All this time as your tenant and this is what you think of me?" I was really gonna give it to him.

But unfortunately for me, I got *that* nurse for my shift. He must have taken a double or something since he usually only worked at night. Just my luck he decided to work extra on the day I really needed to get help. And I needed his help to get prepared and ready for the day. So I was ringing and ringing and I was waiting and waiting and after like an hour and a half, he finally popped his head in. Up until then I didn't realize I had him, and so when I saw his face, I was like, "Oh, no wonder." He just looked at me and rolled his eyes. I was pretty sure that by then he was aware of me reporting him left and right.

I decided I just needed to be direct and give it to him straight. I looked at him and I said, "Look. I have somewhere I *have* to be, and if I miss this appointment, there's going to be H-E-double hockey sticks to pay for. Now all it takes you is five minutes to put me on that machine and roll me into the shower. I can shower myself, I can roll over to the sink, I can wash my face and brush my own teeth, and then I just need you to roll me back into the bedroom and put me on the bed. I can get myself dressed. All you have to do after that is transfer me from my bed to my wheelchair. If you can't take twenty minutes out of your time to get me prepared for what I need to do, then there will *definitely* be H-E-double hockey sticks to pay for."

The nurse, that Norman Bates nurse, just gave me this real sinister look. You could feel it across the room. Just a cold silence and a stare. And then he says, "It's time to catheterize you."

I think I should have been more wary, but at the time, I really didn't care. I was really agitated at the fact that I had him as a nurse again and I was agitated that I had to tell him exactly how I felt in order for him to do his job. I was more aggravated and upset than I was worried or scared. I wasn't cognizant of the danger I was putting myself in by getting angry at him like that. I'm a very easy-going person, but when I get to a point where I'm really upset, I can explode. I shouldn't have exploded on Norman Bates.

The nurse gave me a shot of Lidocaine, a numbing agent, before he did the catheterization so I couldn't feel anything. Then he grabbed about, oh, I don't know how many catheters, but he ended up using six total–and I hate to be so graphic, but I have to at this part–to sever my urethra. There was no need to use six straight catheters to catheterize me. They're small like straws, but one is enough. Any more and it can be dangerous. And while he's supposedly trying to straight catheterize me, he can't seem to figure out where my urethra is. I feel a sharp pain go all the way up my hip and that's when I realize he's doing something seriously wrong.

He said, "Hmm, that's strange. I just can't seem to figure out where this is."

I didn't know if he was lying or telling the truth or what. I asked, "How long have you been doing this?"

"Seventeen years."

"Oh, wow." He must've been taking all that time to hurt me. I'm sure of it. "If you don't know where a urethra is after seventeen years, then I think you need to stop what you're doing, go call the doctor, let the doctor know that you can't seem to figure out where it is, and I'm gonna go finish getting myself prepared to go on my way."

I think I embarrassed him a little after that. He finally stopped and when he walked out, I could feel a trickle. I was so happy because I thought I was trickling on my own. I even said to myself, "Oh, I feel a trickle!"

The rehab aid had started taking care of me and helping me get ready after the nurse left. She rolled me over and discovered what was really happening. I was thinking it was tinkle, but really, it was blood. She saw that and she said, "Oh my, you're bleeding."

I was like, "Whaaa?"

She went to go get the head nurse, and when she came in, she just said, "Oh, that's okay. It's just like a little scab, she'll be all right." They put a Depends on me and got me prepared to go to the courthouse, and the whole time I feel like I'm just constantly going and going and going and going. It didn't feel right. All the way there and I'm just going and going and going. Something was up.

When I got to the courthouse, I learned that I had the wrong court date. I was real frustrated at first, but actually, that mistake was really good for me. If I had been out longer than I was, I probably wouldn't be here to tell the story.

So I was just going and going and going while they took me back to the hospital. I got back to my room and when the rehab aide got there I was like, "Oh man, I'm wet. Can we please get me changed? I can't stop tinkling, I don't know what's going on."

When I changed, my Depends was full of blood. Completely soaked from front to back.

The aide was like, "Oh my God! Oh my God!" She was really freaking out. There was a lot of blood.

I was like, "Well, go get the head nurse! That other nurse did this to me. That Norman Bates nurse! He maliciously did this to me! I asked them so many times not to give him back to me, and he was still here! He did this to me maliciously!"

So she helped me into the bed and the nurse finally came in. There were clots and blood everywhere and the head nurse was like, "Oh, well, you're just having a cycle."

I could not believe her! Did she really think I was okay? I was like, "This is not no cycle. I know better than this. I never bleed like this."

The rehab aide said, "Well, you're going through a change and you probably need a hysterectomy."

"Oh no," I told her. Now they were both trying to explain my injury away! "This is not something I need a hysterectomy for. I know he did this to me, and I told you guys not to give him back to me. And I need to see a doctor."

She said, "Oh, well, you can wait until *the morning* and you can see the doctor then."

"Oh no, there is no way in the world that I'm going to wait until the morning when I'm bleeding like this. Are you serious?"

There were clots of blood *everywhere*.

And then the nurse dared to tell me, "Well, you know, African American people keloid, so that might be what it is."

That was the final straw. I got on my cell phone and I called my friend John. He's the head of the Teamster union. I appreciate him so so much. He picked up, thankfully, and I said, "John, get here quick. I don't know what's happening. They're trying to kill me. I'm bleeding to death and they won't get me medical attention." He told me he was on his way, and as soon as he said that, *then* the aide and the nurse called the paramedics.

The paramedics showed up and they were *livid*. They were so upset about what the nurse had done to me and they knew they had to get me out of there right away. So, naturally, they wheeled me out of there and took me back to the hospital that had punctured my spine. Oh my God, it was a nightmare!

When I got there, I was bleeding so much that one of the nurses almost fainted when she saw me. That's how much blood I was losing. She threw the sheet back over me and walked right on out. Everyone kept coming in to examine me and I kept getting the same expression. They'd just look and cringe and throw the cover back over me. You know it's pretty bad when the medical staff gets queasy. In the medical industry, you're taught to be okay with a lot of blood and fluids and stuff like that. They weren't, so that's when I got even more nervous.

They started asking me these real strange questions. "What is you religion? Do you believe in blood transfusions? Do you have the power of attorney? Do you have a living will?"

I was like, "Why are you asking me all these questions?" I thought I knew why, but I didn't want to accept it. And so I just answered their questions calmly. "No, I don't believe in blood transfusions and no I don't have no living will and do not do this and I'm okay with that and no no no no no."

They got me upstairs, out of the emergency room, and gave me this nurse's aide. I'll never forget it. I've never seen anything like it. I was so tired at this point. It had been such a long day and I just wanted to sleep. But the nurse's aide was sitting at my bedside and she kept rubbing my hand. She was crying, like a little worry cry. And the entire time she was like,

"Don't go to sleep. Please don't go to sleep. Please don't go to sleep." I was just thinking, *What's wrong with her? Can't she just let me go to sleep?*

I was like, "I'm tired. I need some rest. It's been a long day."

But she would not let me go to sleep. Every time I tried to go to sleep, she would keep rubbing my hand and begging me not to nod off.

Now I know exactly why they didn't want me to sleep, and if I'd been in a right mind, I probably would have picked up on it too. But I was drugged up on a heavy pain medication, I was extremely tired, I had had a long day, I'd lost a lot of blood, I had to fuss all day to get where I needed to go, and I just wanted to *sleep*. I thought that by being back in the hospital, I was in a safe, comfortable, warm environment and I could just catch a few Z's while the doctors figured out what they were gonna do. I didn't understand the ramifications of what might happen if I did.

The nurse kept keeping me awake until like one, two o'clock in the morning. I was still up, and by then, I had a doctor–*a doctor*–by my bedside. I had doctors in the emergency room, but to have a doctor at my bedside at one, two o'clock in the morning? Something's wrong. Usually you see the doctors on the floors in the morning. In the emergency room you see them at all times of the day. But for a doctor to be at your bedside in the middle of the night–that's not good.

So he was sitting there and he said, "Miss Rabb?"

"Yeah?"

"I need you to wake up." Man, nobody was letting me fall

asleep!

He said, "I need to talk to you about something very serious. I know you do not believe in blood transfusions."

I was like, "Yeah, you're absolutely right. I don't want nobody else's blood."

I don't know why I didn't want it. I'm a very natural person and if I don't have to do things like surgeries or medications or blood transfusions, I don't want to. Plus there was this big scare about getting HIV/AIDS through blood transfusions a few years before that and I didn't want to risk it. The medical system has that under control now, and I think they had a pretty good handle on it back then too, but I was still cautious. If I didn't absolutely *need* a transfusion, I didn't want one.

"Well, Miss Rabb, I need to tell you that I have blood sitting outside of the room right now of your type. It is really urgent that you take this blood transfusion. I need to explain to you that the body only carries five pints of blood. You have lost over three pints in less than twenty-four hours. And you are still losing blood. We need to replace your blood right now."

I still wasn't sure about it. I asked, "What's the worst-case scenario and what's the best-case scenario?"

He told me, "Worst-case scenario: your organs will dry up, you'll go into a coma, and you'll die. Your organs will completely shut down. Best-case scenario: you live to see another day. Miss Rabb, you can fall into a coma any second now, so my advice to you is to really take heed to what I'm saying."

All I could say was, "Wow."

I didn't have time to call anybody or talk it out or think on it at all. I had to make a snap decision.

I think I was totally freaked out when he told me how dire the situation was. I knew I was sick. I knew I wasn't feeling well. I knew I'd lost blood. But I didn't realize how sick I really was and how much blood I'd really lost. I didn't realize how big a danger zone I was really in. If they had kept me at the Courage Center and made me wait until morning like they wanted to, I would have been dead. So I guess I thought about everything and how major this all was and freaked out. I couldn't call Mom. I couldn't call anybody. I had to make a split second decision, then and there.

So my survival instinct kicked in and I told the doctor, "Okay. Go ahead and give me the blood."

I took the blood transfusion.

I've been through so much malpractice and so much time being sick that sometimes I have days where I wish I hadn't taken that blood transfusion. I would be at peace. I wouldn't have to deal with all the challenges I'm facing. I wouldn't have to struggle anymore.

Those are dark days. And, I'm happy to say, they are few and far between. In the end, I'm glad I took that transfusion, even though I didn't believe in it. By doing so, I could live to see another day and fight to help others like me.

They stabilized me with the blood and had a urologist come in to look me over. Because I had lost so much blood, they thought my kidney or bladder might have been punctured. They couldn't tell. The camera they tried to insert into my bloodstream couldn't make it through because of all my clots, so first they had to flush out all the blood and all the clots just to see what they were dealing with. They wanted to make sure they didn't puncture anything.

So they flushed out my blood while the transfusion was going on and the blood was splattering everywhere—all over the walls, all over the floor, everywhere. They ended up having to give me Norco, which is like the strongest painkiller you can possibly give a person. That was the first time I've ever heard a doctor cuss like that. He was so mad. Oh, he was totally livid. He just cussed right through everything. He was like, "What kind of *F'ing* animal would do some *Shh* like this?"

Next thing I knew, I had somebody come in from Adult Protection Services. I don't know who called them, but they came and said I was a vulnerable adult and I had been taken advantage of. I told them what happened. "Look," I said. "I asked the director of nursing not to give that nurse to me over three times, and he just maliciously severed my urethra on purpose. Who takes six straight catheters to catheterize a person? It only takes one and it's as small as a straw. Can you imagine six at one time? He did this on purpose!"

My health pretty much leveled out after that. I was gonna be okay—or I was gonna be alive anyway. I had to stay in that hospital for a good month or so to get back on point and ready for rehab.

I don't know what happened to that Norman Bates nurse. I don't know if he got reprimanded or if he got fired or if he's still working with them right now with no repercussions whatsoever. I don't even remember his name. But I do remember how horrible he was, and I don't think I'll ever be able to forget the malpractice he put me through. Every time I think about it, I just ask who would do something like that? Who would think that they can just play with a vulnerable person's life like that just because they don't like their job? Just because they don't like the way that person looks? Just because they can?

    That's real sinister.

10 | Escaping Minnesota

After I recovered from that nightmare, no rehab facility in the state of Minnesota would touch me. They said I was unable to be rehabilitated. I think they probably said that because everybody knew about the malpractice that was happening to me and nobody else wanted to get mixed up in it. I tried again with the head of rehab at United but got the same response: "I understand your pain, but you do not qualify for my program."

They couldn't find anybody to take care of me, so a social worker from United decided to just stick me in a nursing home for the rest of my life.

Yeah. Really. I was not about that.

They sent me to this sub-cute nursing home at thirty-nine years old. Everyone there was over sixty, sixty-five. I should not have been there. We had boring peanut butter and jelly sandwiches, Jell-O, and Kool-Aid for dinner, only got showered twice a week, and had "rehab therapy" that was really just the therapists coming in, looking at me, and moving my legs a little bit. No exercise, no nothing. I spent my days in the bedroom by myself. No TV, no nothing. The only TV was downstairs on the first floor. So it was just me sitting there twenty-four seven. And I never saw another patient. I never got to come out to socialize with the other people, never got to go downstairs with the TV, all because I was in a wheelchair and they had such a hard time transferring me–putting me in a wheelchair and getting me down the stairs–that they just left me up there. I'm assuming they didn't have enough staff or time to help me, but that's still not an excuse. Oh my God, I was so depressed.

I wasn't there for long. Not even a week. I couldn't stand it. I didn't know what to do at first, but then my daughter gave me a plan.

She came to visit me one day and I told her, "I need to get out of here. I don't know what to do. I'm going to be stuck here for the rest of my life!"

And my daughter said, "Mommy. Just start rocking. Just start rocking and saying it hurts. They won't know where it hurts, just make something up. Just start rocking and saying it hurts all over. Start moaning. They're going to call the ambulance and we're going to get you out of here. Just keep rocking and saying it hurts."

I couldn't have gotten out any other way. I was signed up for life. So I started making that fake fit. "Oh it hurts! It hurts! It hurts!"

They're like, "What hurts? Where?"

"Oh, it hurts! Everywhere, it hurts!"

They couldn't help me at all so they called the ambulance, and guess where it took me back? United. Of course.

I get back to United and the doctor is really livid with me. He knew instantly that I was faking it. He said, "Miss Rabb. I know there's nothing wrong with you."

I was pleading with him. "I can't go back there. It hurts everywhere. You've got to treat me. I just don't want to go back."

And he said, "Oh, so it hurts huh? All right. We got you."

I would've done anything not to go back to the nursing home. Which included exactly what I was asking for. They gave me so many narcotics–Tylenol #3, Ibuprofen 600, Oxytocin, Naproxen, all of them. They gave me all these pills to try out for my so-called pain, even though they knew I was just doing this to get out of the nursing home. I really didn't know what they were doing. I just didn't want to go back to that depressing place. And my insurance would pay for the medications, so the doctors just went along with it. They almost killed me with all those medications.

During my time back at United, I ran into the infamous rehab doctor again. By this time, I understood that I was never going to get to be in her program. I told her, "You're not going to rehab me, right?"

She said, "Yes, Miss Rabb, now you've got it right. I don't care how many times you ask me. You do not qualify for my program."

So I asked, "Well, what's the best rehab facility in the country? Nobody here in Minnesota wants to rehab me."

The rehab doctor told me it was the Rehab Institute of

Chicago. RIC. When she told me that, I thought I had heard her wrong. I was like, "Did you say Chicago?"

"Yeah, Chicago."

Oooh, I was so excited. I just smiled and said, "Pack me up! I'm going home."

Her eyes got as big as saucers; she was so confused. I had to explain that Chicago was my home. I was from Chicago, and now I was going back. I'd get my rehab *and* I'd be where I belonged.

A friend of mine from Chicago–his name was Thyron–came to visit me after that, but I was so drugged up that I didn't even know he came to see me. He went back to Chicago and contacted Doctor Mack, one of his friends from church and now one of my dear, dear friends. Doctor Mack doesn't work at RIC but she did administrative work in the medical industry and knew a lot of different doctors in the Chicagoland area. He said, "Doctor Mack, you need to get Tonya out of there. They're trying to kill her. She didn't even recognize me."

So Doctor Mack called me. She was talking to me on the phone, but I had a hard time concentrating and talking to people because I was so heavily drugged up that I would fall asleep like every five minutes. I can't believe I even remember my conversation with Doctor Mack. She was telling me, "Tonya, we need to get you out of there. You just find your way to Chicago and on this end I'll take care of you. But you've got to get yourself to Chicago. I can't do anything for you in Minnesota. If you want to go to RIC, we'll make it happen."

Then she asked me, "What is your goal?"

I said, "They said I can't walk again, and I *will* walk again."

That's when I made my mission—my mission to walk.

Doctor Mack got to work. She made some calls and worked on getting me okay to transfer, but United fought her every step of the way. They really gave her a hard time because they didn't want to release me. I think they were scared that if I left, they wouldn't be able to cover up their malpractice anymore. I mean, they were so adamant about me staying that they wouldn't even loan me a wheelchair to get to the airport. Doctor Mack had to order me a wheelchair from Chicago and have it delivered.

Eventually, United did let me leave. What could they do? It was still my choice as a patient. A lot of people don't know this, but you have the right to refuse any procedure or any treatment, as long as you're coherent. Just like when I told them I didn't want the procedure where they punctured my spine. Of course, they still did that one, though. That was definitely an absolute no no. But you have the right to say where you want to be and where you don't want to be, what procedures you want done and what procedures you don't.

My daughter had to get on the computer and pay eight hundred dollars—maybe more—so both of us could fly from Minnesota to Chicago at the last minute. I went to that airport with a folding catheter on and IVs in my arm, looking like I came straight from the hospital (which I did). The airport attendants literally had to pick me up out of the wheelchair and sit me down in one of the seats on the plane, first class too. It reminded me of when I would travel in college.

When we got to Chicago, I was welcomed into the home of one of Doctor Mack's friends, and from there I went to

Rush. RIC didn't have any beds available at the time, and I wanted to try to get a fresh start before jumping back into therapy anyway. Maybe I would get a different diagnosis going to Rush first. Plus, I was excited to be back in the same hospital where I had been as a CNA. They put me in their rehab program and were really working hard with me. I was making good progress. I got all the way to the point where they were having me standing up using the sit-to-stand machine and trying to get me to use the parallels.

You'd be amazed at how many muscles it takes to stand. It takes your quads, your glutes, your core, lots of muscles. All those things work together in order for you to stand. And so you have to do a lot of exercises to strengthen those areas if you're trying to walk again. A lot of the time, they have you strengthen your legs and your core with sit-to-stand and balance exercises. And so doing those exercises makes all your standing muscles work together–from your feet to your calves, to your thighs, to your quads, your glutes, your core, everything that goes into standing.

And once they have you standing, you start doing range of motion activities–ball therapy, the elliptical bike, parallel bars, more sit-to-stand machines, dumbbells and weights. They start teaching you how to do basic everyday activities then, too. They teach you how to roll out of bed, how to sit up on the side, how to put your socks on, your shoes on, all those little things you don't think about until you can't do them anymore. All those things are important too.

Well, one morning after I'd been there three weeks and had progressed so far into the program, one of the nurses was in a hurry. I mean, the staff at Rush was good, better than I remember it being when I was working there, but this particular morning the girl was in a rush to get home and so she was trying to give me my shower really really fast. I was in one of those plastic shower chairs, one of the chairs that disabled people use to stay safe while in the shower and not slip. Well, this one had plastic wheels, and when the shower was finished, she was pushing me out of there pretty fast. Next thing I knew, the wheels got caught on the landing strip between the bathroom and my bedroom and the chair catapulted me out onto the hard concrete floor.

I screamed. Oh, I had no idea what had happened! It was scary. It took about four or five people to get me off the floor, not knowing that I had suffered a hairline fracture in my spine. After the accident, the doctors told me I was having another Devic's relapse and that it was because of the crack in my spine.

They started talking about putting me in a nursing home again and I would not consider it one bit. I was like, "Oh no you're not! I am *not* doing any more nursing homes!" I called Doctor Mack and she told me to call over to RIC and see if they had a bed available for me. I jumped on the phone right away and called RIC. I told them who I was and all about my situation and they gave me like the greatest news ever.

They said, "Okay, Miss Rabb. We've got a bed for you. Come on over here by tomorrow and it's yours."

Finally I was going to the best rehab facility in the country. My mission to walk had just begun.

11 | Professional Patient

It was like a miracle getting into RIC so soon. RIC always has a long waiting list to get in because they're one of the top rehabilitation facilities in the United States. People come from around the world just to go to RIC.

I was extremely lucky. RIC was very beneficial to me.

At first, I was afraid RIC was going to be just like all the other hospitals I'd been to: bad. Anywhere you go, you have good people and you have bad people. I was on a lot of pain meds and really incoherent, and so I slept most of the day except when it was time for therapy. I also had a nurse who was really mean to me. Sometimes she would hurt me when she was getting me prepared for whatever procedure I needed because she thought I was so out of it. I wasn't *that* out of it. I still felt everything.

I have problems with nerve pain, so the slightest touch can

feel so hurtful. The problems started when I started taking Gabapentin at the Courage Center. The meds were supposed to help ease the pain, but really they just made it worse. After I got prescribed them, too, whenever I would complain about the nerve pain the doctors would just up the dosage. It was not good. And so when I got to RIC, they had me at six hundred milligrams, three times a day. They're supposed to take care of your nerves, so if you have multiple sclerosis or Devic's, they administer that to you so it takes care of that sensitivity, but in all actuality, I think it makes things worse because I'd have a fiery sensation that would go through my body and make me scream at the top of my lungs whenever I took it. Each dose would make it get worse, and so the doctors would increase the dosage, and so the more Gabapentin, the more the fire burned through my body. It was one of the worst prescriptions I've ever taken because those medications seemed like they made it worse.

I was having a really difficult time because I was there all by myself. Back in Minnesota at United, my mom wouldn't leave my side. But she didn't come with me to Chicago, and so I was alone. Every time I rang the bell I'd be scared because I didn't know if the nurse who walked through that door was going to hurt me or be rough with me or what. I didn't want to go through what I went through at United ever again.

One thing I've learned about being in the hospital is that you should always have loved ones around you to show the staff that there are people who care about you. If the staff doesn't see that, if they don't see those loved ones, you're just another patient to them, and you can be neglected or harmed or mistreated or who knows what. I always kept my phone charged and in my hands. Sometimes I would just call my mom and make sure she could hear what was going on with me, or I would call my friend in California and make sure he could hear everything that was going on with me, or I would call anyone I knew just so I could have another person there with me whenever hospital staff was in the room. When people would come to handle me, if they were even a little bit rough with me, it would send those fiery sensations through my body and I'd scream. That's why I would always have somebody on the phone. I wanted my loved ones to know how I was being handled when I needed to be changed or cleaned or transferred or anything, and I wanted the hospital staff to know they were live on speakerphone and that someone could hear each and every thing they did. Having those loved ones only a phone call away really protected me during that time.

I think by that point I realized that I wasn't able-bodied. I couldn't push someone's hand away or get up to leave the room or cuss somebody out and tell their supervisor about how terrible they were treating me. I was vulnerable. There was nobody there to protect me. I was scared.

It was always a guess as to who would be coming in to treat me, and so no matter who it was, I always had that speakerphone on. You have some people who handle you kinda roughly but are okay, you have some people who actually care about what they're doing, you have some people who are disgruntled because they feel like they're not earning enough and take out their frustrations on their patients, and sometimes, you have some people who are just maliciously mean. One of those mean people was this physical therapist who would do daily living activities with me.

This lady wrote my rehab plan. It started at the very beginning of a standard rehab plan, even though I had already progressed pretty far at Rush. And she was aggressively mean about me going further. She kept telling me, "Well, you don't qualify to go no further. You don't qualify to go no further. You have to learn how to put your clothes on first. We're not going to do sit-to-stands with you, we're not going to do anything with you until you can get your clothes on."

I kept telling her, "This is a step back from Rush. I need to get stronger so I can stand and walk, not focus on just putting clothes on."

And when I finally showed her I could put my clothes on myself with no problem, she then moved me to this machine where I would have to work my arms until they hurt. She would make me do this every day. It was exhausting. My arms didn't feel like they were getting stronger, they felt like they were about to fall off! I said, "Look, I think you're doing way too much. I think I need time to repair."

She looked at me and was like, "Who are you to tell me how to do my job?"

In my late twenties, I had a brief stint as a bodybuilder. I didn't want all the muscles and everything, I just wanted my body to be in tip-top shape. So I knew a thing or two about working my muscles. I was like, "I used to train. I know the difference. You can't just keep working my muscles like this."

Every session was like a push and pull. She would try to make my program hard, and I would try to tell her she was making it *too* hard. And every night I would call my mom in tears. I would be crying like, "Oh, she's so mean! I just want to be out of here! They're so mean to me! I'm going through all of this and it's awful!"

So here comes Mom to save the day! I was on tons of narcotics and medications and I was just totally out of it. I was sleeping between treatments and therapy and pretty much around the clock, and so one day I'm dozing off and I see this lady walk into the room in a gorgeous red dress, looking like an angel. I saw this fuzzy glow around her and I could've sworn I was hallucinating because the angel looked like my mom. I was like, "Mommy?" And it *was* my mom! She had come to help figure out how to make my rehab sessions better.

I was so incoherent when she came to see me. I was zonked out and everything. Each time I'd nod off she would say, "Tonya! Wake up! What did you take today?"

I was like, "Uh, I took medicine…"

"Tonya! How many milligrams?"

"Um, uh, uh…"

"Tonya! What's the name of the medicine?"

"Um, uh, uh…"

"Tonya!"

She would do this whenever I had called over the phone, too, because she knew something was wrong. I shouldn't have been zonked out like that all the time. So when she came to see me, she talked to the doctor about my condition. The doctor told her, "Well, okay, if she can prove that she can do this, that, and the other thing, then we'll keep her going."

I showed them I was eager to get better and willing to do

the exercises, so they kept me in. They also gave me a new rehab trainer, so I was finally relieved of that mean one who didn't know what she was doing! Things instantly started to turn around for me. They gave me someone else who was *much* better. I was actually really impressed with her because she had a brace on herself. This new rehab specialist had trouble walking too, and so it was like I could relate to her. She understood the struggle of not being able to walk, and she taught me lots of new techniques that really helped my strength grow. She was the one who taught me how to walk again. She would just put my hands on the parallel bars and say, "Okay, I want you to put your torso down, hold your arms on both sides, lean forward and always keep your nose over your toes and push your bottom up and pull with your arms to a standing position." She knew that I needed to learn step by step, and that really helped my progress.

After I finished group therapy, I was finally allowed to go home. I didn't have a home anymore in Chicago, but in order to stay in the rehab program, I needed to live in the city. My daughter was like eighteen at the time and had her own little bachelorette pad in Hyde Park. It was this tiny little studio, but I went to live there with her so I could stay at RIC. The only problem with it was that it had stairs.

When they were releasing me from RIC, they asked me, "Do you have stairs?"

I had already learned that lesson in Minnesota. We did have stairs, but I wasn't about to tell them that. I was like, "No! Nope. I have *no* stairs. None!"

So they let me go.

It was a challenge getting up and down those stairs. I still had to go to therapy and I still had to go to rehab, so I had to make it past those stairs every day. We tried everything! One time my mom and Sha'e even put me on a couch cushion and tried sliding me down the stairs! It was not fun. It was like, "bump bump bump!" That time really hurt my behind!

We didn't have to worry about getting me down the stairs for too long, though. I'll never forget that when I started the day program after getting out of the hospital, there was this guy, Jimmy. He was a transport person for the rehab program and also just a real fun, jolly, upbeat kind of guy. He came to get me one morning and he showed up as my mom and Sha'e were trying to get me down the stairs. Jimmy saw us struggling to get me down the stairs and he said, "Oh, why didn't you tell me you needed some help?" Now, they're not supposed to get us down the stairs because we're not supposed to *have* stairs. They're just an accident waiting to happen. But Jimmy came on over and plopped me in the wheelchair and just boop boop booped me down the stairs. That's how strong he was. He got me down the stairs all by himself! He wasn't out of breath or anything. He was just like, "Let's go!"

Each morning since then, Jimmy would call me on my cell phone before he'd reached our place and say, "I'm en route. You have to be ready when I get there because I'm going to try to keep you on my route. No one else is going to help you down those stairs, so we can't let any of the other drivers snatch you up. I'll make sure to get you where you need to go every day."

Thanks to Jimmy, I was able to get to therapy with no

issues on those stairs and I was getting stronger and stronger day by day.

I went into the day program and I had this really sweet lady. She could tell I'd been through so much. Whenever I was having a bad day, she would stretch my legs and warm me up and she'd try to give me lots of encouragements. She was a real sweet lady. She would walk me around, take me outside, she'd do anything she could to work me and make me stronger. She's the one, more than anyone else, who got me in shape to walk again. She really was.

The day program was also where I went to group therapy sessions. And we had this really cool lady. She sounded like a drill sergeant. She'd be like, "Okay. And one! And two! And three! And four! And five!" And we would do daily activities of living, like moving around in our wheelchair, stretching, mat exercises, the parallel bars, a bit of walking around, all of it. When they finally got us up and walking, they'd try to test how fast we could go. We'd walk as far as we could, as fast as we could, and they'd follow behind with the wheelchair for when we were tired. It was really kinda fun. She would always tell us to go home and do the exercises because they made us stronger–and they really did!

Once I went through the day program, I only had the outpatient program left. They had this awesome guy named Walter–he's still there, actually–and *everybody* loved Walter. He really knows his stuff and cares about his patients. You can't josh with him though. He knows when you're not trying your hardest and he knows when you're not doing your exercises at home and he just knows everything. He can tell where you should be at each point in the program because he's been doing it for such a long time.

I stayed with Walter and RIC for a good three years. They got me up on a walker, they got me up on a cane, and things were really looking good. I was doing really well. Outside of therapy, I'd be working too. My daughter and my mom would take turns walking with me, because in order to recover fully, I had to exercise between therapy sessions. We would go down at night into the little courtyard we had and we'd walk. My daughter would walk me around the courtyard, my mom would walk me around the courtyard, we would walk around the courtyard together all the time.

Sometimes, my mom would force me to go out when I didn't want to. She'd want me to walk, but I wouldn't want to, so she'd just roll me around in a wheelchair. This was all a part of her plan, though, because the sidewalks had a lot of cracks and were so bumpy. My wheelchair didn't have shocks or extra padding or anything like that, so the bumps would hurt so bad sometimes that they would actually encourage me to tell my mom, "Look. Give me the walker and I'll stand up and walk over this bumpy area, and then when we're past it you can give me the wheelchair back."

And of course, once I was up, I didn't want to sit back down. I wanted to keep getting stronger. I guess my mom's plan worked. Those bumpy sidewalks kinda encouraged me to start walking.

I got strong enough to where we were able to move to another place in Hyde Park. The new place had stairs, but they weren't as big an issue this time around. My mom would have me training on the stairs, walking me all the way up the stairs and walking me all the way back down the stairs. We started going on longer walks too.

One time my mom had me walk all the way from 53rd and Maryland to the University of Chicago. I didn't know we'd be going that far beforehand, and I was so upset with her because that's a *long* walk. It's about a whole mile, which might not seem like a lot to someone who is used to walking, but for someone who is just learning how to walk again, it's tough. She just told me, "C'mon Tonya, we're almost there!"

"Well, how much further?" I couldn't see how far we'd gone, thanks to my visual impairment.

"Oh, not that much farther. We're almost there. C'mon Tonya, you can do it. We're almost there!"

And then next thing I knew we're walking across a street. We never walked across the street! I was like, "Mom! How far are we going?"

"Oh Tonya, keep going! We're almost there!"

Finally we get to the University of Chicago and I was out of breath! I was like, "Oh my God." My mom could see I wasn't going anywhere after that, so she sat me down on a bench by one of the university's pools and went all the way back home to get my wheelchair and wheel me back home. It was a workout, and afterwards I was feeling really tired.

When we got back, I was still feeling a little tired, but there were some chores I needed to do before I could rest. We had this big bay kitchen and oh, it was so beautiful! I loved that kitchen. It was the best kitchen I've ever had. And because it was so nice, I liked to keep it clean. I did a lot of cooking–I loved to cook–and so while I was doing all this walking and exercising and getting my strength back, I'd do all that in the kitchen, too. I would go in to cook and have my wheelchair and my walker with me at all times. I'd sit in my wheelchair and then when I needed to cut my vegetables, I'd stand up to cut my vegetables. I'd sit right back down afterward. And then when I needed to put my stuff on the stove, I'd stand up and put my stuff on the stove. And then I'd sit right back down. I knew it was important to walk as much as I could to keep the swelling out of my feet and my ankles, so I'd try to stay on my feet the majority of the day. Whenever I'd get tired, though, I'd just sit right back down.

So when I got back from my super long walk, I decided to clean the kitchen. I rinsed the dishes, put everything in the dishwasher, wiped down the counters, and by the time I was done, I was really tired. My mom said, "Tonya, you need to go to bed." I'd been working so hard, both with the walk and the cleaning, that I was overdoing it. You know how sometimes when you get so tired, you forget where you are and the room starts rearranging itself? I don't know how relatable that is, but I did that to myself sometimes. I'd just work and work and work and work until I drop.

I don't do that anymore though. I learned a valuable lesson.

I decided I needed to take my mother's advice and go to sleep. I told her, "Okay, you're right. I'm going to go ahead and take a shower and then go to sleep."

I stepped into the shower, turned on the water, washed up, and as I was standing there, I was starting to fall asleep. I was so tired that the room rearranged on me and I forgot I was in the shower. I thought I was in the kitchen.

The shower I had was a two-in-one shower and bathtub combo, so in order to step out of it, you've got to pick your feet up. Well, since I forgot I was there, I didn't pick my feet up. I turned to go sideways and suddenly I flipped from standing straight up to falling flat on my back. My head hit the floor—the concrete ceramic tiled floor. It was a big enough fall and impact that I should have died.

My saving grace was this big ol' bun of hair I was wearing on top of my head. It absorbed most of the impact, and if I didn't have that hair, I probably wouldn't be here to tell you about it. There have been lots of near-misses like this throughout my life, I guess.

And so I fell from a standing position to flat on my back. I was crying and crying and crying. I hurt all over. My mom ran in when she heard the commotion and she was so shocked when she saw me on the floor. She was like, "Oh my God! Oh my God! Thank God for your hair." She helped me up and I was okay. I didn't feel hurt, and so I didn't think I needed to go to the hospital. I really was okay.

But then, three or four days later, I started going into total darkness. Another relapse. It was a downward spiral.

When I go through a relapse, the first thing to go is my eyesight. I revert to complete darkness. When I can't see anything but black, I know it's not good. I am legally blind, but my blindness isn't total. I can see a really blurry picture of what's in front of me, but whenever I have a relapse, I see nothing. Total darkness. It's time to go to the hospital at that point. I have to go through all these MRIs, all these CAT scans, and then they give me steroids through an IV for my eyesight to start coming back. And then when my sight is slowly returning, I go to rehab in the hospital, and once I'm through with that, they give me a recommendation to outside rehab therapy programs. Yeah, it's a whole process.

But this time was that my recovery was cut short.

So I was working on recovering from this relapse and I sprained my ankles. I was going to RIC for my rehab program, almost completely recovered from this latest relapse, and on my way home from one of the sessions, I had a cab take me. The ride home was fine and we got there safe and sound, but as I was getting out of the car, there was a high curb. I wasn't in a trained vehicle where the driver knows how to get you in and out safely. I was just in a regular cab. And so as I was stepping out, I didn't realize the curb was so high. It was higher than I was used to, and so I miscalculated my step. I tripped on the curb, afraid of falling yet again on a hard surface. The cab driver tried to help me but he didn't really know how to help me, and so I wobbled and weaved and almost fell completely. There was a guy on the sidewalk nearby who came to my rescue and grabbed me, making sure I didn't hit the ground. Unfortunately, my ankles still got injured. I was rocking around so much that I sprained my ankles.

All that progress in my rehab program, all that progress in recovering from my last relapse, all that work I'd put in to win my strength back, all right down the drain. I was back to square one.

12 | Getting Stronger

I was bed-ridden for a year and a half. I couldn't put weight on my ankles because of the accident, but that injury wasn't the main reason behind my condition. It was just what started it.

While recovering from my sprained ankles, I had to be handled by other people in order to get around. Someone had to transfer me from the bed to the pot and from the pot to the chair and from the chair to the bed each and every day. While I was in the hospital, it was no big deal. The nurses would do it. But when I got back home, I had trouble. My mother wasn't trained in how to move me around. So on one particular day, I really had to go to the bathroom and she was trying and trying to pick me up with all her strength to get me on the pot. She was having trouble with me though. She picked me up, got me to the toilet no problem, but when she was picking me up after I was done going, I accidentally stepped on her foot. She fell, I fell, and she landed right on top of me.

This injury was the worst since I'd fallen in the shower. My whole left side became sprained. I didn't break a single bone, which was good, but sometimes sprains can be worse than breaks, especially when it comes to the ankles. Well, this was one of those instances. I had a huge sprain on my whole left side.

And of course this put me in another relapse. It was the worst relapse I've ever had. I couldn't feed myself, I couldn't clean myself, I couldn't put my clothes on, I couldn't move around, I couldn't do anything. I was back to being totally dependent on others.

We had a big picture window in the living room. It was big and bright and there was always something to watch on the other side of the glass. It was something I'd taken for granted when I could go look out it whenever I wanted. Now that I couldn't walk anymore, I missed it.

So we put my bed in the living room. We turned the living room into my living quarters, no couch, no loveseat, none of the trimmings of a living room. Instead, we had a hospital bed, we had my commode next to that, my wheelchair by the window, a desk nearby that people would sit at when anyone would want to come say hi, and when we got a sit-to-stand machine, that was put in that living room, too. It was literally like a hospital room. My mom took my bedroom.

Every day, I would lay in my bed and look outside that big picture window. There was a space with lots of green grass right next door, and the landlord was nice enough to plant a big rose bush in front of the window so I could look at that while I was bed-ridden. I would just watch those little rose flowers grow each day, and when they finally bloomed, it was wonderful. And when it snowed, all you saw were the roses with snow on the petals. It was so beautiful. Even though I'm visually impaired, I somehow could still see that.

With that beautiful sight right outside my window, I still cried. I looked out of that big picture window and tried to think of peace and serenity and happiness, but it's hard not to cry when you know you can't do anything you used to do and you're solely dependent on someone else to do everything for you. I couldn't feed myself, I couldn't wash my face, I couldn't get out of that bed, I couldn't do anything by myself. It's a lot of work for one person to care for you twenty-four seven. For me, that was my mother. It was way too much for her. Way too much. Knowing she had to take care of me all the time just made my situation even more depressing. It took every ounce of me not to give up. It would have been easy for me to, but after being through so much already, I knew how important it was to stay positive. I had to make a plan.

I started drinking smoothies. I wanted to try to heal my body by quitting solid foods. It would be easier for me to eat (or drink, I guess) at my own pace and digest everything properly. My mom would blend my herbs, my fruit, my juices every day for breakfast and lunch, and then for dinner I would have warm soups all blended up. They were actually pretty yummy! Everything I ate I pretty much drank through a straw because I couldn't feed myself. I also didn't like how whenever someone would feed me—my mom, mostly—they would always be impatient, being all like, "Hurry up! Eat your food quicker!"

As I started to get better, I wound up going back and forth to the hospital almost every month. You name it, that's what I was there for. Relapses. New catheters. More medications. Checkups. Colds. Everything. I'm serious, I was there for everything. In and out and in and out, three times a week.

One of those medical appointments I had to go to was to see a neurologist again. I have always been unsure of my diagnosis. I believe I've had a lot of things happen to me over a long period of time. I don't know what exactly is wrong, but I know there's *something* not right with me. I'm just doing it one day at a time, and so when I started going through these relapses again, I decided to pay a neurologist another visit. I went to a neurologist at Northwestern who was a specialist in Devic's and they said, "Oh, well you probably don't have Devic's." I was shocked. I was excited. Maybe I didn't have this disease that for years I'd been told I had.

They took like eight or ten vials of blood from me that day and I left. When I came back for the results, the doctor who had been real sharp just a few days before had her head down and wasn't looking at me in my face. I knew exactly what she was gonna say before she even said it.

"I'm sorry to give you this news. You do have Devic's."

I said, "Hold on, you told me when I came in the other day that I didn't have Devic's. You told me the Mayo Clinic said I was okay!"

She just said, "Well, the Mayo Clinic made a mistake."

Oh, I was like totally disappointed. Totally frustrated. They had my hopes up and then they just came right back down again.

The neurologist then started telling me about treatments. "You have a few options," she said. "You can undergo this chemotherapy treatment, you can take this medicine that may cause brain damage, or you can take this other medicine that may cause leukemia." It was pretty much like they were telling me, "Either way you're going to die, but we might as well try to do something preventative to help you last a little bit longer. So which one would you like to try?"

That was a hard pill for me to swallow. First and foremost, the doctor had been confident that I didn't have Devic's. She was assertive and looked me right in my eyes. She knew what she was talking about. But then when I came back, she did a total flip-flop like there's this hypocritical oath doctors make so that they never ever go behind each other's backs and say one of them made a mistake. They always back each other up. That's how I think it works. When one doctor makes a mistake, they all just fall into line and go with it. And with the wonderful World Wide Web, it's harder for someone in my position, someone who is a patient, to start all over because your records follow you everywhere. They're all computerized. It's hard to get away from malpractice because it just keeps following you.

So basically the neurologist had given me a choice: chemotherapy, brain damage, or leukemia. Chemotherapy can wipe you out completely. Leukemia is nothing to play with. And even if I'm basically just a brain in a jar, all I have left is that brain, so why would I jeopardize the only thing going for me? There was no good option.

I ended up telling the neurologist, "You know what? I'll

take my chances. I'm not gonna do any of them."

I went back home after that and I prayed. I prayed a lot through all these journeys and whenever I had extreme pain, and I prayed after they had given me all these grave options too. I was scared. I said, "God, I've been having a really rough time. Please help me through this pain. Let me have a day where it doesn't hurt so bad. They don't have a clue what they're doing. Give me the wisdom of how to heal myself. Please help me and guide me through this."

Praying helped me through the worst of it. I started going to therapy at Warren Barr and I was getting stronger. I was getting better. I was also leaving the apartment more and more, and that meant I had to deal with one simple obstacle I never thought I'd have to deal with again: stairs.

Now, before the last series of accidents, I hadn't anticipated on going backwards, and so I didn't really think twice about the stairs anymore. Once I lost my movement, though, oh, those stairs were a pain! We had to struggle with the stairs again every time I needed to leave the apartment. My mom couldn't get me down by herself, so we became totally dependent on the fire department. My mom would get me dressed for the day, we'd call the fire department, and some firemen would come to get me down the stairs. They'd leave and we'd sit and wait at the door for the handicapped cab service to come and get us. It took a little longer than it used to, but we made it work.

The only time the fire department is supposed to come, though, is when you're going to a medical appointment. But I still needed to get groceries, and my mom couldn't go out to get them herself. Even though she takes care of me, I take care of her, too. We do everything together; we're like a partnership. We have to be. And so in order for us to get in and out of the apartment, we had to tell the fire department we were going to a medical appointment each time we called them, and then somehow we would have to sneak over to the grocery store instead of going to a medical appointment. Eventually the fire department caught on because we were calling so often. They knew we had to eat, though, so they didn't make a big complaint about us going to get groceries. I am so grateful for the fire department. I know they had bigger emergencies to deal with than just getting me down the stairs, but they were still kind enough to help me in my time of need. I am so, so, so grateful for them!

There was such a massive effort behind making sure I could get to therapy each day. Everyone involved was instrumental in my efforts to getting strong again. I went to therapy at Warren Barr for almost a year and a half. But I just wasn't getting strong enough quickly enough. It was like I was learning everything all over again. They were trying their best to rehab me but I was just in so much pain that they couldn't do much.

I wasn't making enough progress in the program so I was discharged from Warren Barr. I went back over to RIC, hoping they'd be able to help me. They gave me like three sessions, and then the worst thing that could have happened, happened.

My insurance tapped out.

I didn't have the money to pay for any more sessions. I think it might've even tapped out before then and they were just taking pity on me. I can't remember. All I know is that without insurance, I wouldn't be able to get back to where I was.

I became really sad and depressed. I didn't know how long I would be in that totally dependent state. If I didn't continue to work on getting stronger, I'd be that way forever. I couldn't have that.

I went to RIC and was like, "Well, if my insurance ran out and there's nothing you guys can do to help me for six months, what do you think I'm going to be like in six more months with no therapy? I won't be able to use any of my muscles or anything!"

They were like, "Well… um…"

And then I asked them, "Can I pay for more therapy sessions in cash?"

They said, "No, Tonya, you can't pay cash. You don't have the money."

"Well, can I go and get some more insurance?"

"No, Tonya, you can't go get any more insurance. It just is what it is."

"What can I do then?"

They were like, "You can go to the RIC gym and you can pay a personal trainer to do practically what we do. You can pay for water therapy treatment with someone else and you can use our facility. But we can't let you back into our program for another six months."

But I couldn't make that happen. I looked into water therapy treatment but each session was fifty dollars a piece. Physical therapy with a personal trainer was like a hundred and fifty dollars an hour. When I was in the program, I was getting both of those with my insurance. I couldn't afford it without that insurance, but I was out until it reset after six months.

I went from getting therapy three times a week to doing no exercise whatsoever. That kind of change for someone who is on the road to recovery can be drastic. I didn't know what to do. I have this determination, though, like an internal mechanism that just keeps me going. Whenever I want to quit, something inside me doesn't allow me to. I just keep going.

So this obstacle was just one of many. When my insurance ran out and I ran out of options, I told myself, "Okay, well, I can't go to rehab no more. What am I gonna do? I know! I'm gonna start a nonprofit called 'Tonya's Mission to Walk' and I'm gonna put up a website where my friends and family can go to donate. I'm going to pay these personal trainers to help with my therapy and I'm gonna do this water treatment at RIC and I'm not going to give up. Failure is not an option!"

At first I only really got donations from close friends, and it was like totally random at times, too. One friend would be like, "Oh, I think you need some new shoes, so here's a care package!" Or another would be like, "Here's some money for this or that or whatever." Or another would be like, "You need some entertainment! Here are some movies!" It was really just a collaboration of everyone just trying to pitch in with what they could, when they could. I didn't really raise as much as I needed to, but it was a start.

Without being able to really move, I was like dead weight. I was entirely dependent on other people. So when it was time for me to leave, they wanted to put me in a nursing home.

Now, I have this fear of the nursing home after my last experience with the one in Minnesota. I was *not* going to go back to a home. My mom told the doctors, "No, she's coming home with me."

They told her, "The only way she can come home with you is if she has a sit-to-stand machine with her Hoyer Lift that can help you transfer her from the toilet to the bed and visa versa. You're not trained to move her otherwise."

Oh, it was like I had a mission then! I called around to different companies to see how much a sit-to-stand machine would cost and where I might be able to get one. I called company after company and everyone's like, "Yeah, this automatic Hoyer Lift with a sit-to-stand machine costs twenty grand, fifteen grand, ten grand," and so on and so on. Different prices all around, but still all out of my price range.

With each company I was like, "Well, can you take a payment plan?"

"Nope," they all told me. "You got to pay for it upfront."

I finally found one company who was willing to work with me. I was like, "Look. I have this nonprofit called Tonya's Mission to Walk and I have several people who have pledged to pay for this machine on a monthly basis. Is there any way we can set up a payment plan with me and six other people to pay for this over a couple of months?"

And they told me, "Yep, we can do that." I was so ecstatic. Their kindness allowed me to come home with my mom. It was a total blessing.

It was a sit-to-stand Hoyer Lift, meaning it would force me to stand up and my mom could easily roll me over to wherever

I needed to go. At the same time, it was making me stronger because it would force me to stand up and work those leg muscles. And I had this all because of those few but generous donations from family and friends.

I had been through so much, and after this small success, I had a newfound determination. I didn't want to give up. I was like, "I refuse to be a part of the system! I'm not going to give up and I'm going to fight fight fight fight to the very end! I *will* walk again!" And so even though I didn't get too many donations from that initial campaign, I got a Hoyer Lift out of it! It was the start of something that I wanted to expand.

Those donations were the start of Tonya's Mission to Walk. It was *my* mission to walk at that point, it wasn't what it is today, but it was a start. The idea had started to take hold.

13 | Tonya's Mission to Walk

When I became bed-ridden after those relapses, I did two things. The first thing I did was start that small fund for the Hoyer Lift that has since then grown into Tonya's Mission to Walk. The second thing I did was visit a naturopath.

A naturopath is a doctor of natural medicine. A doctor who uses herbs to heal people. A friend of mine had referred me to one, and so I went to see what he was all about.

The first thing I noticed when I met Dr. Christian were his long silver locks running all the way down from his head, just like mine. He was an older gentleman in his eighties, but he looked like he was in his forties. It was one of those Helma B type deals! He introduced himself to me and then he was like, "Okay, we're gonna start with some deep breathing."

So we're doing the exercise, breathing in and out all slowly and deep, and I asked him, "How's this gonna help me?"

He explained, "You half breathe, half live to get your chi going. Let's do this!" So he helped me with the breathing exercises and then he was like, "Okay, now we're gonna stretch."

I was still wondering how it was gonna help me. But then I was amazed that I was able to stretch and move without having spasms. It didn't hurt like it usually did. We did that all in our first session.

I paid him for the first initial visit, and he opened my eyes to alternative medicine. The only problem was that the doctor was so expensive–his services were like three hundred dollars a month. I couldn't afford it.

Oh, but he was so kind to me! He saw that I was in real bad shape and said, "Look, Sweetie. My herbs are really expensive and I know you can't afford them, but I'll do whatever I can to give you advice over the phone. You have to follow my instructions to a T though. The day you decide you don't want to listen, the day you don't want to follow my instructions, I cut you loose."

I was so happy. I was like, "I'll do anything to get better!"

Dr. Christian was a different kind of doctor. He would need to have an update each day–either he'd call you or you gotta call him–but you had to talk to him every day. He's got to know what's going on with you and where you are health-wise. You'd be in touch with him so much that you couldn't josh him. You might tell him, "Yeah, I'm doing everything you're telling me to do," but if you're still showing symptoms, he'd be like, "Okay, so if you're doing everything then why do you still have this symptom? What are you eating? What instructions aren't you following?" He'd just know. Over a period of time you figure out which foods do what to you and how your body reacts each time you try different things, and he'd guide you on what your diet should be like.

I gave up solid foods to drink smoothies instead when I started learning from Dr. Christian. What a lot of people don't realize is that a lot of diseases start with your diet. When doctors say that diseases are hereditary, sometimes it's because you pick up your eating habits from your family. Everybody eats the same dishes, everybody likes the same foods, and so therefore, everybody shares the same nutrients. Your disease *becomes* a hereditary disease through that same diet. And so in order to get healthy, you've got to start eating healthy.

And that's the hardest part! Oh, it was so tortuous to kick all the foods I'd been eating since I was a child. I was like, "What? No dairy? Are you serious? I need cheese! I need milk! Dairy is its own food group! What do you mean I can't have pizza? What kind of game is this? What do you mean I can't eat potato chips? I love potato chips!"

Those snacks were the hardest things for me to kick, but I was *really really really* sick. It was either I went with what the traditional medical system was going to do for me–which, remember, was them saying they couldn't treat me and that I was going to die and so I needed to just take whatever experimental drugs they wanted to give me and deal with the side effects–or I could start doing something preventative through making changes to my diet and environment. I'm pretty sure there was only one right answer.

Doing it naturally is a long, drawn-out process though.

You have to change the way you eat, you have to take your herbal medicine, you have to drink your teas, you have to breathe evenly, you have to meditate, you have to do all these things you're not used to doing. So it's a long, tiring, hard process. If it takes you a long time to get sick, it's gonna take you a long time to get well.

I couldn't handle it. Dr. Christian eventually cut me loose because there were just certain things I couldn't get away from. Like the occasional Snickers bar or the bag of potato chips or the slice of pizza from Domino's–things that weren't healthy for me. You can send your body through a lot of shock when you're used to eating a certain way and then completely switch things up all of a sudden. It has to be a gradual process, and Dr. Christian's process was too fast for me.

When he cut me loose, I was really scared because I could feel some of his stuff working and I didn't want to lose that progress the same way I'd lost my rehab. I was like, "What am I going to do now?" I stuck with my smoothies and some of the healthy eating and I got this idea: Why not pay to go to school and learn all this alternative medicine for myself? Why not help me and my family for generations to come–and other people as well–with this knowledge? I decided I wanted to learn more about naturopathy. I decided to go back to school for Eastern Asian Medicine.

Oh, that was a challenge: going back to school after six years of having graduated already. I settled on going to Pacific College of Oriental Medicine, right here in Chicago. When I showed up and they saw me in a wheelchair and they saw that I was visually impaired, people didn't know what to do! I think people are naturally afraid of what they don't understand, and when they first meet me they're not quite sure what to think. One of those people who didn't take too kindly to me was this admissions guy who was very unprofessional and very insensitive. I went to him to sign up for school and he started talking to me in that way people do when they realize you're blind: trying to enunciate and speak up because they somehow think you can't hear either. "I want to UNDERSTAND if you can SEE well enough to see WHAT I'm SAYING and MEET the REQUIREMENTS because YOU are BLIND."

What was ironic about it is that in Eastern Asian Medicine, there are quite a few doctors who are completely blind. Sometimes they are the best acupuncturists or even herbalists because their senses are more sensitive. They know what an acupuncture needle should feel like when put into your skin or what a certain herb should smell and taste like.

I think that director just didn't want to let me into the program. He gave me all these different requirements that didn't even make sense. Like, he said I needed to be able to pick up sixty pounds to be in the program and a bunch of other stuff that had nothing to do with what I would be learning. I was really disgruntled because he was making up all these stipulations so that I couldn't get into the program. I had a really high GPA, really good transcripts from all my past schooling, and they still didn't want me. I was hurt.

I just said, "Well, if I can't go to this school to study Eastern Asian Medicine, I'll go to a different school, or I'll go to school for Public Administration or something other than Eastern Asian Medicine to write policies and rules for people with physical challenges who are less fortunate. People like me."

Oh boy, Tonya was on a mission. I was on a mission to help everybody and anybody. I was like the poster child for trying to walk again and being visually impaired and overcoming physical challenges. I still am! And so I was ready to make my next move.

DeVry had a program for Eastern Asian Medicine, and I went there for a semester. Their accommodations for disabled students, however, weren't up to par. Their professors were great and I learned a lot, but unfortunately, I couldn't keep up with the work because I wasn't getting the help I needed. I was failing.

Luckily for me, I got a call from Pacific College of Oriental Medicine, the school that I had been originally denied from because of my disability, while I was going through these problems with DeVry. The new director–I don't remember her name–told me, "Look, we got rid of that jerk who kept you from enrolling. He no longer works here. I'm the new director and I'm going to bring you into this program. We see that you have a high GPA, we liked your submission for the program, and we're more than willing to work with you. Why don't you come on back?"

And so just like that, I left DeVry and went to PCOM instead!

Oh, I was so excited! I think they fired that guy because of his noncompliance of the Disability Act and how it says if a school is accepting money from the federal government, they have to make reasonable accommodations for those who are physically challenged or disabled. They can't turn you away because of the disability. They have to make some accommodations for you. And I think once they found out what that guy did to me, they cut him loose. I don't know what happened on their end, and I don't really care. I was just excited to be going there!

I started getting acupuncture done, I started learning about herbs, I started learning more about my human anatomy and how things were associated with my illness, I even learned about my mother's health and her heart issues. I think over the period of time where she was trying to take care of me, it probably put a lot of wear and tear on her body as well, and so I was able to help her with this new education.

There were lots of professors who were really awesome and went the extra mile to make sure I stayed in the program. They saw that I was trying my best and they were willing to help. But it was still a rough start at PCOM. After the first quarter, they tried to tell me I was failing a majority of my classes. I was like, "Nah, that's not possible! I'm a straight-A student, I'm working hard, I'm studying—why would I be failing?" We had to have a sit down to discuss what was going on and what extra accommodations I might need. We were talking about different options when I said, "Well, I'll tell you what. What if you give me a tutor for each one of my classes, and so that way if your tutor fails, we know something's definitely wrong." They liked the idea, so I got a new tutor.

I started pulling better grades from my classes. It was practically A's and B's (and maybe a C here or there). I was pulling it off. I was putting in a lot of hard work and dedication, spending like eight hours a day, five days a week at the school working on my studies, both in class and in tutoring. I was working harder than most of my classmates because that's what I had to do. That's what I'd been doing for most of my life.

I knew that because of my challenges, I had to work extra hard. As a person with physical challenges, I had to do things differently. I had to do things more slowly. In order to compete with the normal world you have to invest a lot of extra time, and so where it might take somebody an hour or two to do something, it may take me four to six hours to do it–but I'll get it done. So in order for me to stay in this program, I went to class two days out of the week, but I was at the school five days a week, eight hours a day, studying and working and being in tutoring. All that just to get a good grade, or a semi-good grade, in most classes.

I would get good grades in most of the classes, but in one particular class, the professor wouldn't give me the grade that I deserved. There was one incident where I had a take-home final test, and I went above and beyond. I answered all the questions exactly how I was supposed to answer them, full of the right facts and figures and everything like it's straight from the textbook. I turned it in and then instead of getting an A or a B, the professor gave me a C minus.

I was shocked. I thought I'd done so well on it. I went to his office said, "Let's go over this test question by question to see if you can tell me how I got C minus from an A paper." He said okay and we started going over the answers and he was nodding his head and everything like I was getting the answers right.

Once we were done, he was like, "Oh yeah, that was a really good read actually. It's quite educational, lots of information. But I didn't discuss most of that in class."

I was like, "Okay, this is totally unfair." If I put in all the right stuff, what did it matter if he didn't discuss it in class? I just didn't get it.

The school stood behind him. But I understand his perspective. I was going above and beyond and was fighting my way through this program because it was helping me stay alive. That was the only reason I was there.

I think it's important to share the struggles I've faced even with the accommodations I've had during my schooling because having those accommodations doesn't just make everything into a bed of roses. The extra help I get doesn't put my ability over those who are able-bodied. It just levels the playing field–and most times I'm still at a disadvantage! I probably deal with a whole lot more physical obstacles every day than the average person does in a week. I'm not even mentioning the challenges I face as a woman, or the ones I face because of my race. I have so many layers and layers and layers of challenges: I'm a woman, I'm black, I'm blind, I'm in a wheelchair. I have a lot of strikes against me. Some days it can be very challenging because I'm tired of the challenges, but I still have to wake up every day and put my best foot forward. Whenever I'm in the biggest funk I just say, "Okay, this sucks. I've got ten minutes of sulking and then I've got to get up and keep moving." I've just got to keep moving. Life isn't just what happens to you. It's twenty percent of what happens to you and eighty percent of how you deal with it. I choose to deal with it head-on. I choose to overcome those challenges I have.

Especially because I'm one of the lucky ones whose physical challenges are visible. You have people who are walking around every day with challenges you and I can't see. We all have challenges that we have to work through, and I think it's important to remind people about that. Just because you can't see someone's challenges doesn't mean they aren't there.

I think it was this mindset that kinda got me going on the nonprofit. After going to school for Eastern Asian Medicine, my health started to improve. I didn't have to go to the hospital all the time, my symptoms started turning around, and I started getting stronger. I still had my physical challenges, but they weren't as debilitating as before. In fact, I hadn't been to the hospital in over three years.

And so as I started getting stronger, I started focusing more on what I could do for others like me. I still had the website up and I said, "You know what? Why be selfish and only collect money for my own needs? There are other people out there who are probably going through the challenges that I'm going through, so why not try to help them?"

That was the beginning of Tonya's Mission to Walk. I decided to take the website I already had and add a Facebook page to reach more people. Then I started thinking about everything in my life and how I could bring it all together so that I could use those experiences to help others.

One of those experiences was the gap in my insurance. That challenge was honestly one of the biggest I've faced because there was nothing I could do about it. And so that's where I started with Tonya's Mission to Walk. I wanted to help bridge the gap between insurance collapses for those who have no other options. We have funds and programs to help those people so they don't have to try to stress about figuring it out and starting all over again.

We also are helping with expired equipment. Technically, you only qualify for new equipment every five years. If something happens before then, oh well. There's nothing anybody will do for you. I found out about that policy and I was just livid. So Tonya's Mission to Walk has an exchange program where if you or your loved ones have equipment that is no longer in use, you can donate it to the program and it will get to someone in need. Maybe that's someone whose chair stopped working or maybe that's someone who may need a walker *and* a wheelchair but only qualifies for one.

In addition to that, we're currently working on bringing in technicians for automated wheelchairs to help keep your chair properly maintained. Maybe you don't need a completely new chair, you just need yours fixed up. We got you.

What I've discovered through my journey is that there isn't a lot of accessibility for those who really need it. It's hard to create normalcy for someone who is physically challenged. It's almost like you have to be really wealthy to live a comfortable, normal life when you're dealing with physical challenges! I want people to be able to maintain that normal lifestyle that is hard to maintain when your life isn't normal. That's what we're here for. Tonya's Mission to Walk is as much a nonprofit with various programs as it is a community of people with challenges, a support group for people struggling with their health. We'll share stories, share cautions, share tips, and we'll make a friendly, positive community for each person in our network. We just want to help people reach a point where they can be fashionably challenged, and you can own your challenges and make them a part of your own style. It's not a disability. It's a characteristic.

That good support system is part of your healing. And basically with this nonprofit I wanted to create a cycle of healing. I believe in healing economics. I have always thought that you can honestly do good and help people and make an earning while at it. Having caring economics is a win-win situation.

With that healing cycle, I wanted to expand to help even those who aren't physically challenged, and I separated that into four different groups: youth, professionals, veterans, and women.

I've always been an advocate for our youth. So we've got the Youth Growth connection. I believe children should have a chance to grow, and a part of that is through arts education. They don't have music and arts in school like they used to, but it is really important to have that artistic space because it allows you to use both sides of your brain–which is really important in learning. And those programs are after school, where kids are most likely to get caught up in trouble and whatnot. If the youth don't have something positive to occupy their time after school, they'll get into trouble. So why not come to Tonya's Mission to Walk?

I'm also an advocate for those who have retired. These

professionals are so full of wisdom and knowledge and after they've done such a good job for twenty, thirty years, they retire and all that knowledge is gone. Why should that wisdom go to waste when a retired professional could mentor a young teen? That professional could teach that teen a valuable trait so they can have a jumpstart toward a career where one day they can reach back and teach a teen, too.

I'm also from a family full of veterans. It's a military family. One of my uncles who I love dearly just retired as a colonel. He was really influential to me during my childhood. He would always mentor me and spend time with me like I was his daughter. I really look up to him and I'm very proud of him. He went into the military at seventeen and he just retired at fifty eight, so he spent pretty much his whole life in the military, and to watch a person dedicate so much of their life like that is inspiring. We may not always agree on the reasons why we have to go to war, but we all have loved ones who are putting their lives on the line, and that decision affects our lives. When they come back they may be battered and wounded and might not even be the same person we knew, but they sacrificed themselves to make sure that we would be okay back at home. Being so close to a loved one in the military, I noticed that there are a lot of veterans who come back and just don't know what to do. Why not make a program with Tonya's Mission to Walk where we can highlight that veteran's honor and help them keep their integrity? We can provide services for them as well, training them how to help with rehabilitating those with physical challenges or rebuilding homes to be more wheelchair friendly or utilizing their computer skills to help with our online programs. We can help veterans with whatever help they might need.

The fourth category is women. I'm a woman, so why not help other women like me? Simple!

I took all the challenges I've faced over my lifetime and said to myself, "When you see a need, you fill it." I took all the challenges and malpractice I've experienced as a patient, I took all the challenges I've experienced when I had to give up my cosmetology profession, I took all the challenges I've experienced as a student, I took all the challenges I've experienced as a person with loved ones in the military, and I took all the challenges I've experienced as a woman, and I bundled that all up into one big cycle of healing. Why not build something where everyone can help each other and heal each other and make their community grow?

Tonya's Mission to Walk is not just about people who want to walk. Tonya's Mission to Walk is all about extraordinary people with extraordinary challenges. So whether you're visually impaired or you're not able to walk or you're going through other challenges that are just as important, that's what we're here for. We're here to help.

This memoir that you're almost done reading is meant to share my story and help introduce the world to what we're doing here at Tonya's Mission to Walk. I want people with challenges to live their life with dignity and pride, and I want Tonya's Mission to Walk to be the support system that helps people through their challenges. We're not where we want to be yet–we're just starting out–but we're on our way. Right now we're looking for professionals who can help train volunteers and build out our programs. We're looking for drivers to drive, we're looking for technicians to help out with equipment, we're looking for therapists to host group therapy sessions, we're looking for anybody who's ready and willing to help our cause. Most importantly, we're looking to be a positive difference in people's lives.

Just because you have challenges doesn't mean you have to stop living. You can still have a career, you can still be married, you can still have children, you can still go out for an evening on the town, you can still be glamorous, you can be anything you want to be. You don't have to live your life lonely. You don't have to be forgotten. You don't have to be left behind. I have been through pretty much everything. If you're going through something hard, I know how you feel. I know you're hurting, and I know you're tired of all the challenges. But I want you to know that it's important to stay positive. I've been through so many challenges with my health and with my career and with my schooling, but what keeps me going is this nonprofit. All my life, I've figured there's a reason behind my challenges, and I think this is it. This nonprofit is how I make a difference on the world.

Be active in your health. Don't put your life in someone's hands just because they say they're a professional. Have a loved one nearby, both when you're in the hospital and when you're not. Always take notes. Always ask questions. Ask, "What's the best-case scenario? What's the worst-case scenario? What are the side effects? Will I eventually be happy with this choice?"

Don't be afraid to seek out training. Don't be afraid to ask around and find out what you can do to make your life a little more comfortable.

Learn how to smell the roses. Learn how to smile and laugh. Learn how to treat yourself. Know that it's okay to cry if you need to cry. That's part of healing too. It's okay to have a day where you just don't want to be around anyone. It's okay to have a day where you just want to be around everyone. Live every day like it's your last and be grateful for everything you have. Gratitude is a great attitude.

Don't give up on yourself. No matter what you're going through, we all hit out peaks and valleys. Do not give up on yourself. You are important and you are here for a reason. You are here to touch somebody's life, even if it's just one person. And again, don't give up on yourself. That one's worth repeating.

When I first lost my vision, I thought my life was over. But it wasn't. My life kept going, and I think the most important lesson I've learned is that life doesn't stop after blindness. Life doesn't stop after any challenge.

Life still goes on. No matter your outlook, it continues. I choose to be positive. I believe we can do all the things we put our mind to, and that we can overcome any obstacle, no matter how big. I believe in extraordinary people with extraordinary challenges, and I believe that when we have obstacles in our way, we don't stop doing things.

We just do things differently.

Epilogue | Just Doing Things Differently

I was born a healthy child. I had twenty-twenty vision, was athletically inclined, ran track, did marching band, trained to be Miss USA in bodybuilding, went to school for journalism (for a hot second), worked in spas all around Chicago, did makeup for the Industry, went to business school, got married, had a child, suffered from heartbreak, lived a fully-lived life all before I became blind. If I hadn't lived the life that I've lived, I would think I was lying.

I had gone through three careers–seventeen years in the beauty industry, eight to ten years doing makeup for the entertainment industry, and then back to school for business– by the time I lost my vision. Three careers. And with the latter part, I learned how to continue on with a sudden disability. I got strong enough to go *back* to school.

You'll be amazed by what you can accomplish. *I'm* amazed at what I've accomplished. You can do anything you put your mind to. It may take longer. It may be more of a challenge.

You may have to go the extra mile to be recognized, but at the end of the day, you can do anything you put your mind to.

So where do I go from here? I don't know for sure. I do know, however, that I will never give up the thought that I might possibly walk again. If I don't get there, at least I'll know that I put one hundred and ten percent into that mission.

I think I might want to marry again. I might want to travel. I think I might want to have my own wellness studio and I think I might want to open wellness resort one day. I think I'd like to help people build their businesses and help them start new ventures. And, of course, I want to keep growing and keep expanding Tonya's Mission to Walk. That's pretty much a given.

Basically what that all boils down to is that I don't plan on slowing down. I'm just going to keep doing things differently. I'm going to take life one day at a time, and one day I might be completely healed again, but if not, I'll still be completely healed in my own special way.

Acknowledgments

My grandmother told me once that if you can count on one hand how many true friends you have, you are a rich person indeed. She also said that there are good people out there and it's your job to go find them.

I am so appreciative of the following people, all of which fall into those two categories. I can never say thank you enough, but right now I'd like to try.

Miss Dorris for your love and support. May you rest in peace.
Steven Deer for molding my beauty career.
Marshall and Tyra for giving me my start as an artist.
Chad Bowe for being my rehabilitation counselor and giving me everything I wanted and more, even when you weren't supposed to. Thanks for also helping me get those A's!
Dewey Miles for continual support.
Senator Betty McCullom for ensuring I had the right to walk across the graduation stage.
Michael Hill for opening many doors for me.
Anil Lewis for showing me that blindness is a characteristic, not a disability!
Eduardo for helping me learn Spanish.
Mr. Battle for being an awesome mentor.
Dr. Singleton for giving me the pathway to the keys to prosperity.
Jawar for introducing me to *Breaking Into the Music Industry 101* and for believing in me.
C. Ward for your support and patience.

Doctor Mack for being a great mentor and friend.

Emily for teaching me how to do things differently.

Walter, **Khan**, **Cody**, and **Francisco** for being super therapist extraordinaires!

John Kobler for supporting any and all of my outrageous ideas, and especially for being a great friend. Ryan is always in my prayers.

Bill, **Dave**, and **Theseus** for making sure I always have a smile on my face and for showing genuine concern whenever my mom and I step out that door.

Mr. Breelin for my journey to Sapelo Island and also for being a great mentor.

Dr. Laurent for showing me that I can be a gracious leader.

Julie for sharing her experience and going the extra mile as a professor to make sure I succeed.

Sheldon Smith for sharing your knowledge and wisdom as a millennial with me. Continue to do great things with the Dove Tail project!

Mrs. Booth for seeing something in me as a little girl to pick me out of one in a thousand. You're the greatest drama teacher ever! (Emerson Performing Arts school)

Cornbread Harris for showing me my circle of fifths and being an awesome friend.

George Burns for giving me my first business and showing me a taste of independence.

Dr. Nobantu Ankoanda, edu for being a great activist and mentor.

Folami for being a beautiful, sweet spirit.

Ayanna for being the same and consistent at all times.

Zuzu and **Jonathan** for your support and love.
Lawrence for being so awesome and totally capturing my personality!
Colonel David Rabb for your many years of service and mentorship, and for showing me the importance of diversity and inclusion. You are greatly appreciated!
My grandmother for helping build a solid foundation for me. May you rest in peace.
My sister. You know who you are!
My daughter, for trying to be the best you can be.
My family, externally and internally, because sharing is caring and love is the most important thing of all.
Last but not least, I want to thank **my Mommy**. Hopefully she won't get mad at me calling her that!

A special thank you to the organizations who have helped me along the way: **National Federation for the Blind, Center for Vision Loss, BLIND, Inc., State Service for the Blind of Minnesota, the Shirley Ryan AbilityLab (formerly Rehabilitation Institute of Chicago, RIC), National Seating, Future Business Leaders of America/Student Government Association (Herzing University), the AMBCC, Student Senate/MnSCU (Metropolitan State),** and **University of St. Thomas.**

Everyone who has made a difference in my life and supported me through my journey, I appreciate you all! Thank you, thank you, thank you!

About the Authors

TONYA RABB is the founder of Tonya's Mission to Walk, a Chicago-based nonprofit that supports "extraordinary people with extraordinary challenges" through a variety of services. Learn more about Tonya and her nonprofit at **tmtowalk.com**.

LAWRENCE SILVEIRA is a writer and editor from California. See more of his work at **writerlawrence.com**.

www.ingramcontent.com/pod-product-compliance
Lightning Source LLC
Chambersburg PA
CBHW031620210526
45464CB00004B/1671